NO SUCH THING AS A
DIABETIC!

Kirrily Chambers

Published by Kirrily Chambers

ISBN: 978-0-6457183-0-0 (paperback)

First edition, 2023

For book orders and enquiries,
contact: kirrily.chambers@gmail.com

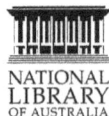

NATIONAL
LIBRARY
OF AUSTRALIA

A catalogue record for this
work is available from the
National Library of Australia

Acknowledgements

There are so many individuals I must thank for this book who without them not only would the book not have been written but I would not be the person I am today.

My family: To my mum and dad for giving me the strength and courage to stand up for myself and to always have the confidence to ask loads of questions. To my brother and his family who no matter how many times we bicker I always know you are there for me. My Aunty Trish who has been my support growing up and after the death of both my parents.

To my family that are not actually related to me but certainly are my family (in no order): Mark and Vicki, Bill and Nicci, Alex, Tamara and Paul, Jayne who has always supported my career amongst other things, Megan and Steve, Lynn (and Andy), Mags, Lisa, Trish and Laz, Kristen and Chris.

And to my health care team who do more than just look after my health care needs in a very nonjudgmental way but who I truly respect and consider friends: Dr Tony, Dr Toby, Dr Phil, Dr Mark, Toni, Tim and David.

Contents

Introduction

Being asked by Kirrily to edit her book was great honour – and quite a challenge!

Kirrily begins her story as a child when, freshly diagnosed with type 1 diabetes, her life becomes filled with a myriad of questions. Kirrily, the adult writer, finds herself unable to leave you, the reader, in the same state of confusion, so uses her knowledge as a Credentialled Diabetes Educator and Pharmacist to explain many of the more complex issues. You will find these throughout the book set in italics.

Kirrily's story is at times startling, occasionally sad, but always extraordinary. Through it all shines her zest for life, her refusal to give up – yes, a stubborn streak! - and her over-arching resilience which continues to leave me in awe.

This is the story of a person who has scaled mountains, the size of which would daunt lesser mortals; has traversed the deep and dark valleys of life which the rest of us fear to imagine; and who truly knows the value of cherished friendship, and indeed, of life itself.

I hope you are able to hear the authenticity of Kirrily's voice as she tells you of her remarkable journey.

Lynn Bonython

CHAPTER 1

Triskaidekaphobia

I am not superstitious by nature. Admittedly I don't walk under ladders but that seems just common sense. Black cats crossing my path don't faze me and I have always been careful with mirrors but only because I really don't want to clean up the mess if one gets broken! However, triskaidekaphobia, or the irrational fear of the number 13, fascinates me. The fact that owners of hotels and tall buildings avoid the use of numbers just so they do not need to address the number 13 due to superstition is so interesting!

It is not known where the fear of the number thirteen originally came from but there are many theories. Some believe it is because Jesus had a last supper with thirteen followers and Judas, who is believed to have later betrayed him, was the thirteenth disciple. Others believe it comes from Viking culture. It is thought Loki, the 13th God of Norse mythology, was the 13th guest to arrive at the funeral of the god Balder whom he had murdered. This may be where it became a superstition for number 13 to be unlucky.

Triskaidekaphobia may be the reason I remember my blood glucose level at diagnosis of my type 1 diabetes. It may also be because I have a good memory (or so I have always been told).

13.6 mmol/L. The magic number.

The blood glucose reading for someone who does not have diabetes is roughly 5.5 mmol/L before the first meal of the day [known as fasting] and 7.8 mmol/L two hours after food.

That number and what it would subsequently mean would change not only my life but my family's life and, in the years to come, shape the way I relate to food, my friendships and relationships, my self worth and ultimately my career and acceptance of who I am and what makes me unique.

My childhood is filled with wonderful memories. Growing up in a reasonably large country city, my brother and I got to experience what I believe to be the best of both worlds. We were raised in Port Lincoln, a city in the lower Eyre Peninsula, approximately 646 km from South Australia's capital, Adelaide. It is in Boston Bay and is surrounded by swimming beaches, surf beaches and lucrative fisheries.

We had weekends of swimming and all sorts of water sports as well as camping trips, motorbike riding, fishing and lots of outdoor sports and games. We did still have the use of most "city" facilities, albeit small and limited. There was shopping and fashion (although not what would rival the large cities or catwalks of the world), plenty of places to eat and even a movie theatre open on weekends! Having recently been back to Port Lincoln and seeing advancements and changes that have come with growth, I am pleased to see it has kept the country charm while being able to keep up with progress.

One of my fondest memories from childhood is that for two weeks every year we would go on family holidays. Nowhere fancy because my family was not wealthy but that does not matter to a child. What matters is time spent with your Mum and Dad and your big brother, enjoying each other's company and, even back in those days, being away from the rat race of having to be somewhere at a certain time. What I remember most about family holidays is how relaxed my parents were! We would often rent a shack in Coffin Bay about 30 minutes from Port Lincoln. Other years we would take the caravan to Wallaroo, a small town on the western side of Yorke Peninsula. It was for those two weeks each year that we would have extra treats and soft drinks that we were not allowed during the rest of the year.

However, things started to change for me and my family when I was about 8 years old. I would often have severe stomach pains, for no clear reason and with no diagnosis or cause. One such instance ended up with me in the Port Lincoln hospital delaying our departure for our annual family holiday to Wallaroo. The reason? Unknown. Having spent overnight in the Port Lincoln Hospital undergoing several blood tests and scans, the doctors were at a loss to determine exactly why I was in agony with extreme stomach pain less than 24 hours earlier yet feeling fine the next day! They sent me home, and my family and I were able to go on our holiday after all.

Other occasions would include admissions to hospital for episodes of delirium caused by prolonged elevated temperatures and febrile convulsions. As a child I remember going to the Women's and Children's Hospital for scans to check for epilepsy due to the convulsions and being in an enormous room (it would have been enormous for a child!) with loads of stuffed toys. I had had several severe convulsions for no apparent reason, so again at a loss to find a reason for my bizarre symptoms, the doctors in Port Lincoln wanted further investigations. I remember not being able to play with any of the stuffed toys due to needing to remain perfectly still for the CT scanner. Really?? That seemed mean, making a child sit perfectly still and not allowing them to play with anything. The result of the scan, however, was no epilepsy and again no reason for the seizures, just maybe the result of high temperatures.

I also remember as a child having Mum question me about a large bruise on my arm and asking how I got it. I had no idea and really, how important is that in the scheme of things when you need to be thinking about who you are going to play with after school and what is for dinner because you are hungry!!? Oh, ok back to the GP. This time it was different. This time blood results revealed something "odd". Now we must go to a physician.

A physician is different to a general practitioner. Physicians are GPs who have studied for longer in a chosen specialty in order that they have extra skills to diagnose and treat complex medical conditions. As an adult, I now have an enormous respect for the stress and worry that these two years of not knowing would have placed on my parents, yet I was completely oblivious to how they must have felt at the time.

However, two visits to the physician later, still with no diagnosis and no answer, it was just the "wait and see, come back if symptoms reappear" game.

So, despite numerous trips to doctors and hospitals being almost part of our routine now, January 1983 started like any other family holiday. Two weeks in Wallaroo in our caravan in the caravan park. Wallaroo is a town on the Yorke Peninsula 160 kms north-northwest of Adelaide and one of my favourite holiday destinations as a child. This again may have been because despite being lucky enough to have grown up in a city that is situated on the coast and being exposed much more than the average child to the beach, holidays here and in Coffin Bay meant every single moment in the water. Despite hot days and nights with no air conditioning in either the family car or caravan, I loved seeing lots of family friends, young and old.

The second week in January 1983 however was tiring for me. I had no energy, was thirsty much more than normal and was getting up frequently in the middle of the night to walk all the way to the community caravan park bathroom. The second last night of our stay I was so tired, I wet the bed! Oh, my goodness, how embarrassing! How could I ever tell my Mum, especially if my brother found out!? My Mum however was great (as she always was) and told me not to worry because "these things happen" ("Not to me they don't!" was my way of thinking!!).

Often when driving back home to Port Lincoln, we would stop at Whyalla (described as the third most inhabited South Australian city) to visit my Mum's sister and brother-in-law. This time due to the heat, Dad decided to stay overnight and finish the journey home the next day. The irony of only being allowed soft drink and sweets as children on special occasions and two weeks of holidays does not escape me now as an adult. I still have distinct memories of watching a video of "Ghost Busters" and drinking a two-litre bottle of Coke within half an hour but still being thirsty. I was extremely uncomfortable, not being able to quench my thirst. Having to ask for more to drink suddenly alerted my parents that there might be something seriously wrong with me. Great! Another trip to the doctor!

So off we went to a GP in Whyalla. By that time, I really did feel incredibly unwell, so I did not argue. It was here the doctor first did a urine glucose check, followed by a blood glucose check. I remember while waiting for these results, my Mum commented that she suddenly realised how much weight I had lost! Then the unforgettable number! 13.6mmol/L.

Blood glucose levels are measured in millimoles per litre of blood (mmol/L); a mole being a scientific unit of measurement often used to measure chemicals.

The female doctor told my Mum I had juvenile diabetes (now known as type 1 diabetes). She asked Mum if we had any diabetes in the family. My maternal grandmother had type 2 diabetes, but this is not at all related, even though they are SO often confused.

What did this mean? According to this GP (and I will be kind because it is such a long time since I was first diagnosed) this meant (as she explained to me) no more ice cream, sweets and treats and soft drinks! Forever!

What she told my Mum was that I should have nothing to eat or drink until I got home to Port Lincoln (some three hours' drive if we left immediately) and I should then be taken immediately to the Port Lincoln hospital where I would be admitted as she was ringing ahead to let them know we were coming. Wow, how dangerous we know that to be now! With not enough insulin being produced and my body not getting any energy from my food meant fat and muscle quickly started breaking down. The by-product of fat breakdown produces ketones which can be a serious consequence for people with type 1 diabetes at diagnosis and when they are unwell (amongst other times).

The information we were given when I was first diagnosed was the best knowledge the medical professionals had at the time but boy, the outcome could have had a very different ending!

The 3-hour trip home was torture. Not having any real under-standing of what the diagnosis of diabetes meant, and like many of the general population having seen someone on medication that causes a low blood glucose level, or a hypoglycaemic episode that requires glucose, I wondered what "type" of diabetes I had. Did I have the "type" that could not eat sugar or the other "type" that "needed" to eat it? What was going on? What did it all mean and why did I have to go to hospital? I also remember wondering if I could still do "normal stuff" like go to university (something I had always wanted to do) and play sport. The two consolations of that trip were that Mum sat in the back seat with me all the way home and Dad didn't get cross with me when I asked him to stop because I needed to go to the toilet (a pet hate of Dad's on long trips!). Such simple consolations for a ten-year-old!

Arriving at the Port Lincoln hospital and having been admitted began the learning curve every individual and family are faced with upon diagnosis of type 1 diabetes. When asked by my Dad during visiting hours a couple of days later how I felt, I remember answering him with an honest " Like a pin cushion!". Having arrived in the "children's" ward of the awfully familiar Port Lincoln hospital, I was soon hooked up to an IV with some insulin and started on a monitoring of hourly blood glucose levels. This meant a nurse coming into my room every hour or so and pricking my finger to draw blood to see how much glucose was in my blood before consulting some "magical empirical equation" that calculated how much insulin I should be given that would bring my glucose levels back into a range that is considered healthy (years later I understood this to be called a sliding scale).

At this point, having had no real input from any medically trained individuals, I still had no clue what everything was about or even if I would ever be "normal" again.

From the next two weeks as an inpatient I have some amazing memories of slowly starting to feel better and some beautiful, compassionate nursing staff who helped me, as a ten-year-old child, get my head around this extraordinarily complex health condition. Interestingly I would never look at an orange the same way again! The skin of an orange offers resistance similar to human skin so on Day 6 of the hospital stay I was given a syringe and an orange and was told that these were mine to practice with before I gave myself my own insulin. Pin cushion anyone?

At ten years old I was obviously too young to question or refuse what I was being told or asked to do because I never questioned or asked why or refused any of what the doctors, nurses, or Mum or Dad required, told, or asked of me.

The learning curve was steep. Food, something I had not really thought much of before now required A LOT of thought! What was a complex carbohydrate, a refined sugar, a fat, a protein, let alone how much each serve was "worth" and whether it would or would not affect my glucose results was SO much for me and my family to take in. Probably obvious to me as an adult but a burning question to me as a child was does toothpaste have sugar in it and did I need to "count it" in my daily allowance of food? BUT I was blessed with intelligence, common sense and was a quick learner. So, here's what I learnt (and remember this was a long time ago):

Everything we eat, regardless of what it is, is used as energy. Our food is broken down as sugar (or the correct wording is glucose) and moves into our cells (of which we are made up) where we can use it for everyday living. To understand the way the body works, we use the lock and key analogy. Insulin is a hormone that is produced in the pancreas which is the key that unlocks all the doors in our cells to allow the glucose (broken down in our stomach from our food) to move from our blood. Without keys, the sugar (or glucose) builds up in the blood and symptoms (like blurred vision, frequency in urination, feeling tired all the time and thirst) occur.

Type 1 diabetes is an autoimmune condition. What this means is the body wakes up one day and decides it does not like the cells that produce insulin and "kills" them. What causes this is not really known. There are many theories including the clean gene theory. The result is no insulin (or keys) to open the doors.

The clean gene theory (among many others) stems from the fact that type 1 diabetes has had a dramatic increase in numbers in the 20th century.

This may be in line with better living conditions (humans now have sewage etc.). What might be also consistent with this is our gut biome are less regularly exposed to bacteria and viruses to allow our protective micro-organisms to flourish. It has been proposed that removing the microbial "filth" in our everyday lives may somehow have a long-term consequence on our health.

Type 2 (or what used to be called mature age or late onset) diabetes often gets confused with type 1 diabetes, although more than forty years ago it was not all that prevalent. The way this is described is that while individuals will always produce some of their own keys, these keys are faulty and are not made in enough quantity. In majority of those diagnosed with type 2 diabetes, there is also putty in the keyholes (fat) which is why there is a significant emphasis on weight management as part of health. While tablets are used in the early stages of type 2 diabetes, this is a progressive condition, and it is often necessary to prescribe insulin to keep individuals healthy. There is very much a misconception type 2 diabetes "can turn into" type 1. However, this is not the case. The autoimmune process must occur for the diagnosis of type 1.

Obviously at age ten I learnt an exceedingly small much more simplistic version of this lock and key analogy. It was not until years later when I became a health professional that I became much more interested in how the body works and how insulin and food are so intertwined. However, what my family and I were taught to survive during these two weeks stay in hospital was this:

1. Inject a mixture of short and long-acting insulin at breakfast and tea every day (this regimen of insulin was all that was available when I was diagnosed, unlike now where we have "smarter" insulin)

2. Eat a certain amount of complex carbohydrates foods (such as rice, pasta, cereal, and bread) at breakfast, morning tea, lunch, afternoon tea, tea, and supper in an attempt to keep glucose levels as stable as possible throughout the day and night.

3. Match what you eat to the physical activity you do all day. This includes day to day living and sports and physical activity. Does anyone know exactly how much energy is "burnt up" in any one activity in any one-time frame??

4. If you get it wrong, your blood glucose levels could be above target (high glucose levels, called hyperglycaemia and you will feel like crap).

5. If you get it wrong, your blood glucose levels could drop below target (called hypoglycaemia and you will feel like crap).

Most individuals will tell you hypoglycaemia or "hypos" (low blood glucose levels) are what most individuals with diabetes (regardless of what type) all fear most. Not only do they make us feel horrid, but symptoms can also be challenging and frightening. The feared nocturnal hypo which occurs in the middle of the night when you are asleep is also one of the most difficult psychological aspects of diabetes management.

Reasons for hypoglycaemic events include too much insulin, increased physical activity (including exercise), not enough food, hot weather, changes in skin temperature, varying injection technique, alcohol, a combination of some or all of these, and sometimes for no apparent reason at all.

Symptoms include shaking, sweating (a cold rather than a warm sweat like when for example you have been running) numb extremities and mouth, confusion, nausea and less commonly, unconsciousness.

Before leaving hospital (where I wanted to stay because this was where I now felt safe surrounded by health professionals who I felt knew what they were doing!) the health care team decided that it would be beneficial for me to experience a hypoglycaemic episode so I would be able to recognise symptoms in the future. Upon reflection years later, while I still agree with this practice, I certainly do not agree with how my first hypoglycaemic episode was executed!

Individuals who are diagnosed with type 1 diabetes are often recognised to have what we now call a "honeymoon period" when they are first diagnosed. What this means is usually lower amounts of external insulin is required to be injected during the period soon after diagnosis. How long that period lasts is very individualised.

For me, though, there was no honeymoon period after diagnosis! I learnt exceedingly early in my diagnosis that my body would never really "follow" any rules. Years after studying health, I now wonder if the couple of years of questionable symptoms before diagnosis reflected above target glucose levels and my body's reactions to them. Perhaps that was my honeymoon. So, with no honeymoon period while in hospital it was unlikely that my symptoms would develop as the health care team expected. What this meant was that I did not "behave" as expected when the "planned hypo" began!!

Viewing the supposed interesting "experiment" (bearing in mind that type 1 diabetes was very uncommon some forty years ago) were my GP, my physician (ironically the same one I saw for my bruise), nurses, my Mum, my Dad, my brother and probably many people I do not remember. So given the known causes of hypoglycaemia, (too much insulin, physical activity, heat, not enough or delayed food, etc) I was instructed to administer my breakfast insulin (the orange was very relieved!) and breakfast was withheld. Everyone expected the hypo to then occur. Nope! Nothing happened. No hypoglycaemic episode. Odd, really, because the textbooks said that insulin plus no food equals an immediate hypoglycaemic episode. And of course, the textbooks are ALWAYS correct, right?? It would take me years and lots of training to understand the pharmacokinetics of the older insulin.

Pharmacokinetics means the activity of medicines in the body over time including how they are absorbed, distributed in tissues and excreted from the body.

The supposed "short" acting insulin we had access to years ago really is not all that short acting at all and can take quite some time to work. While I know and appreciate that now, the health professionals looking after me and expecting me to "behave" in a predictable way did not. No hypoglycaemic episode equals my fault, right? It would have to be my fault! What other possible explanation could there be? So now the health professionals had to do something else! Extra insulin required. Great, another insulin injection and more waiting while everyone in the room continued to watch, wait, and stare at me expecting me to do I am not exactly sure what! A couple of hours later still no hypo! What else causes hypoglycaemia? Physical activity. So now a nurse and I were walking up and down the hospital corridors. This really is something years later I remember quite well!

Fast forward an hour: still no hypo. Now the nurse and I were running up and down the stairs. Still no hypo.

Fast forward another hour. Finally, after nearly four hours of people staring at me, I started having symptoms of a hypo! Sweating, shaking, feeling hungry, nauseated, emotional (although translated for a ten-year-old that meant feeling like you wanted to cry). Ok, good, now I know what my symptoms are, can I have my breakfast?

NOPE

Apparently, the physician decided what would be a good idea was to get the ten-year-old to tell him about the EXACT treatment for a hypo. After all, this was the reason for the morning's exercise was it not? To get me to understand and experience my symptoms and know how to treat them because this would keep me safe in the future! However, the brain becomes starved of glucose during a hypoglycaemic episode so trying to recall anything is difficult. I do however recall being yelled at when I was unable to clearly define how many jellybeans I should eat when I was experiencing that hypo. Fortunately, the GP present had some sense and started giving me some sugar mixed in water (jellybeans are MUCH yummier but sugar will do the trick. Yelling, on the other hand, does not). While my recollection of this as a ten-year-old may not be as precise as some of the adults in the room, my parents have confirmed that these events did indeed happen as I have told it.

Welcome to hypos! Welcome to diabetes!

CHAPTER 2

Structured Routine

There is very much a misconception that insulin is a cure for type 1 diabetes. If you are diagnosed with type 1 diabetes and inject your insulin, then things will be fine, right? While this is some of the story, it is not all of it. The primary goal of anyone with diabetes is to maintain glucose levels as close to target range as possible. Having learnt in hospital to inject the orange and obviously myself with insulin, among many other things I also had to learn to do blood glucose readings a minimum of twice a day. This involved pricking my finger with a small needle (called a lancet) and obtaining a small sample of blood for a machine (called known as a glucometer, or blood glucose machine) to analyse.

Over the years and as a health care professional, I have come to realise that twice a day is not nearly enough times to monitor how often my glucose levels may be within range and have increased this to sometimes up to and exceeding twenty times a day.

Years after becoming a health professional, I learnt Ames developed and introduced paper strips called Dextrostix in 1965 to help those diagnosed with diabetes measure their blood glucose levels. You added a drop of blood to these strips, waited 60 seconds and then washed the blood off with water. A result was determined by checking the colour of the strip against the colour chart. Before this time individuals diagnosed with diabetes monitored their glucose levels with urine strips. While better than nothing at all, it has long been recognised that blood monitoring is more accurate and more time sensitive than urine analysis. In 1970, realising that the Dextrostix were difficult to use, a scientist by the name of Anton H. Clemens invented a meter that reflected light and gave a reading (in the form of a swinging needle). The name of this first meter was the A.R.M. (Ames Reflectance Meter) and it used the same Dextrostix that had been used for several years before!

This meter however was large and cumbersome and had problems in that the battery was made of lead acid. And so began the race to develop small more user-friendly meters and bring them to the market. In the mid-70s a German company Boehringer Mannheim developed a competitor glucose strip called the Chemstrip BG (it took them another six years to develop a machine to read these strips, but this meter has now been recognised as the original Accu-Check meter). In 1977-1978 Boehringer Mannheim also sponsored an international symposium called "Diabetes in the 80s" which explored the idea of home glucose monitoring. This revolutionised the way the current market felt about the machinery currently available. This moved forward the concept of meters being more compact and user-friendly and the Ames third generation meter, called the Glucometer was developed.

And so, armed with this amazing new technology some forty years ago, I was released from hospital with my insulin injections and my new (very difficult to use compared to today's standards) home blood glucose monitoring equipment.

These home monitors were not "portable" and were the size and weight of a house brick (which is why twice a day morning and night monitoring was recommended). I do remember a meter before this one pictured that required rinsing off the blood using water from a water bottle supplied with the kit!

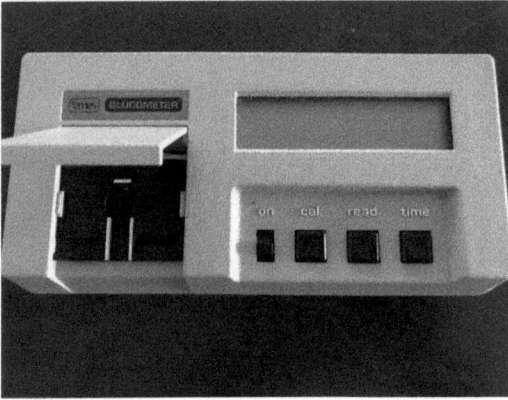

Special thanks to Joanne Taylor for the use of the image.

The lancing devices were not much more user friendly than the meters but again in those days, the devices were only just coming available for home use. It is interesting to see how far technology has come, and not knowing any different, I accepted that this was now my new "normal".

And so, began my (and my family's) strict and structured routine.

Insulin is required for everyone, even when we are not eating which is why I was required to inject both short and long-acting insulin. My childhood routine started at 7am with a blood glucose reading, then a mix of short and long-acting insulin, then my breakfast half an hour after my injection. From this injection in the morning I was committed for the rest of the day to eat regular amounts of complex carbohydrates at regular times (morning tea at 10.30 am, lunch at 1 pm, afternoon tea at 4pm) followed by a second blood glucose result and mix of the short and long acting insulin at 5:30pm and more regular amounts of complex carbohydrates at regular times (dinner at 6pm, half an hour after the second injection for the day and supper at 9pm). This regular routine would, in theory, result in very stable glucose levels, which was the ultimate goal for me, and it still is for anyone with diabetes.

So, no sleep ins, no early nights because supper MUST be adhered to, to prevent the nocturnal hypoglycaemic episodes that could occur. Sick days were an absolute nightmare. I was given tablets (on prescription which years later I learnt were prochlorperazine) to "prevent vomiting at all costs because vomiting causes glucose levels to drop low and if unable to eat this would be a huge problem". The huge problem really is it is exceedingly difficult to stop someone vomiting when the body wants to! And again, it is not that simple, as vomiting and having no food in your stomach does not automatically mean low glucose levels.

Sick day management of type 1 diabetes (and the knowledge we now have years on) shows stress has an enormous impact on glucose levels so they may indeed fall or perhaps rise, depending on circumstances.

Nonetheless we, as a family, learnt as much as we could from the health care team of doctors and dietitians and changed our lifestyle. We substituted simple sugars (lollies and "normal" cakes etc) for diabetes friendly cakes (made with artificial sweeteners) and ate regular carbohydrates. I religiously injected my insulin, participated in blood glucose monitoring, and had regular checks with my health care team. Provided I did everything I was "told" my three-month glucose level (known as a HbA1c) would be within target. Right? Ummm not quite! No matter how much I worked at my glucose levels and how hard I tried I was never able to produce the magical HbA1c number of less than 7% (or thereabouts). Not that I really understood all these numbers. I was, after all, just a child.

Interestingly, again as a health professional I was taught at a university level one of the most important things that I can do for an individual with any chronic health condition is to empower them. Perhaps this is a new concept but asking me to monitor my glucose levels twice a day (standard protocol forty years ago) and then not giving me any skills to make any changes based on these random numbers made the exercise meaningless. No individual, let alone a child, will do this short term, let alone long term if there is no clear purpose for it.

I was to "present" the "evidence" of my monitoring to my physician once every three months so that I could be told there was clearly something I was not "doing right" for the glucose levels to be "so high all the time", and "things needed to change."

I do remember my mum preparing meals and counting the carbohydrates with me into 10-gram amounts. One portion in those days was 10 g and all complex carbohydrates eaten had to be weighed and measured and allocated portions (1 portion = 10 g). I still remember the allocation of portions for my day; 2 portions (20 g) for breakfast, 1 portion for morning tea, 3 portions for lunch, 1 portion for afternoon tea, 6 portions for dinner and 3 portions for supper. This did not take into account salad, vegetables or protein and made some days difficult to eat anything else but carbohydrate. Always the same amounts of carbs to ensure my blood glucose levels were stable throughout the day.

I was always regularly active throughout my childhood, both before and after my diagnosis. I played both summer and winter netball, was a runner in school and involved in interschool sports every year in high school. Sports days for me were interesting. Before and after every sprint I had to drink a glass of unsweetened orange juice to prevent me hypoing. Hard to run when you are participating in 7 events for the day (14 glasses of orange juice anyone?).

I am incredibly lucky to have had amazing parents who did everything they could to support and nurture me. I recall one night at

5:30pm sitting at the table staring at my syringe but telling my Mum I did not want to do my insulin anymore. Her response was "Ok, get in the car." When I asked her where we were going, she told me we would have to go up the hospital and find a nurse to give me my needle and that this was what we would have to do twice a day for the rest of my life if I didn't want to inject. It did not take me long to pick up my syringe, mix my two insulins and inject into my stomach! Admittedly I remember not liking her very much at the time. Years later, after becoming a health professional, I have come to realise the incredible balance between nurturing and discipline it took as a parent to allow me to develop and grow as a child who would be able to look after myself with a chronic health condition.

Despite the nurturing, despite having no refined sugar and the strict unwavering regimen, I was unable to achieve that magical HbA1c number of 7% or even come close. In fact, I was unable to even achieve blood glucose levels that did not bounce from below target to above target and everything in between! On a very personal note, every month, or thereabouts two days before my period was due, I would have glucose levels that would skyrocket and then the night before my period, I would have severe hypoglycaemic episodes often in the middle of the night.

When I asked my physician about this, he told me there was no relationship between the two!!!! Of course, we now know better and have much more ability to help individuals negotiate the relationship between hormones and fluctuating glucose results.

I was extremely fortunate to be able to go to "diabetic" camp when I was about 12 years of age. These are still run today around Australia and the world and are designed to build self-esteem, confidence, and self-management for children with type 1 diabetes. I remember going to Victor Harbor, a small coastal town about 80 kms south of the city of Adelaide. There I met many kids my own age all with type 1 diabetes but having all being diagnosed at different ages. It was fantastic to connect with children who were my peers and feel "normal", where injecting insulin, monitoring blood glucose levels and having a hypo were all considered "normal". While the camp also helped my self-esteem, there were some other beliefs I stumbled across that I was unable to comprehend immediately and took some time to accept, especially from an emotional perspective.

One of the concepts I had been taught at diagnosis was I must never, never, never eat simple sugar (unless I was having a hypo) because then I might end up with complications! This is one of the scare tactics sadly still being used in some practices today. Being told to never eat chocolate, cake, sweet biscuits, and lollies again may have worked for a while but as humans, it is in our nature to question and challenge. To give my Mum the credit she deserves, she did an exceptional job of sourcing "yummy, almost unable to tell the difference" recipes and cooked some amazing food. And please remember this is before the invention of such things as stevia and other sweeteners that do not actually disintegrate when exposed to high heat.

However, at diabetes camp, suddenly surrounded by kids my own age, all with type 1 diabetes, not only did I learn that I really was quite "normal", I also learnt that if I ate simple sugar in the form of lollies and chocolate I wouldn't suddenly die (or of course, immediately develop horrendous complications that the health care professionals had been threatening me with!) Oh sure, I would have an above target glucose level, sometimes outrageously so, and I would feel crappy for a couple of hours, but I wasn't dead, was I? At about the age of 12, I began to question everything I was told by the supposed "experts". The reason? They had lost my trust.

Fortunately, learning that I could eat refined sugar was not the only thing I learnt at diabetes camp! I also began to learn that rigid doses of insulin need not be adhered to when being super active.

Canoeing was fun, especially with lots of kids my own age, although there were pauses to treat many hypoglycaemic episodes along the way! AND did I mention how "normal" I felt? How great is peer support! I felt "normal" for the first time since diagnosis! Sure, I learnt that I could eat refined sugar and rebel occasionally and that I wouldn't suddenly die! However, more importantly, I learnt I was the one who had ultimate say over how I would manage my condition because it was my body. I learnt how to adjust my insulin doses depending on how much physical activity I was participating in and how much food I was eating and that I did not have to stick to a set amount of insulin every single day. It was here at camp I learnt that it was ok to stand up for myself and tell the "experts" (insert the word doctors) that they did not necessarily know everything about my diabetes. I actually had a say in this because it was my body and while I was still learning about my diabetes, they could not just dismiss my opinion!

So having spent three (or maybe four days) at camp, home I went with renewed faith in MY OWN ability to manage my diabetes. That faith lasted maybe until the next HbA1c result and the subsequent "telling off" by the health professionals. I simply could not understand my results. I would religiously inject, religiously monitor, and religiously eat everything I was told to eat. Yet often I would go to sleep with a glucose result well within target and wake up the next morning way above target! How did that happen?? According to the supposed "experts" it was me sneaking food in the middle of the night. That would explain it, right? After all I was a child and there could not possibly be ANY other explanation. Um, wrong again! Years later we now know about something called the Dawn Phenomenon. Hormones released between the hours of 2am and 8am increase insulin resistance and cause exactly what I was experiencing. However, I was told off instead! My fault again! Back to the doctor to be reprimanded.

On one such occasion, that I remember well, I met Mum at the physician's rooms after school on a Thursday afternoon. Bracing myself for another dressing down, I was not disappointed. Having been told the latest HbA1c was completely "unacceptable" I was then handed a strict diet. Looking back now this diet was very much a low glycaemic index regimen and very much ahead of its time.

Knowing much more about diabetes and the relationship it has with food, we now use food and food groups much more as treatment for chronic health conditions. Carbohydrates are not all equal and we now know some have slower (low GI) influence on glucose levels compared to high GI (faster) influence. Low glycaemic index foods have a value less than approximately 55 and are slower absorbed, digested, and metabolised. They cause a lower rise in blood glucose levels (and keep us fuller for longer) and therefore require smaller amounts of insulin.

And so, began a multigrain bread, baked bean, and lentil diet. Ok, not that bad. In fact, I would love these foods now, except baked beans. I have never liked baked beans! Nonetheless as a teenager, I was not so keen on any of it. However, I had been told to change my whole diet so change it I did. For four days!

I do not think even the physician who suggested the radical change in food had any understanding of the magnitude of difference to my blood glucose levels this would make. Over the course of the four days, slowly but surely my glucose levels started to decline. However there had been no adjustment to my insulin doses. I remember going to bed Monday night having spent some time sitting in the passage of our house talking on the telephone to one of my classmates about a project for year 10. The rest I must rely on accounts from my Mum and brother, and later my father who was at work as the incident all unfolded.

Mum tells me I woke up on Tuesday morning and behaved as normal. I went into the kitchen and injected my insulin as usual, half an hour before breakfast. Then I went to have a shower. Mum says about 10-15 minutes later she began yelling at me to get out of the shower because I was using too much water and would be late for school. Having yelled at me a couple of times with no answer, she stormed into the bathroom. She recalls me standing unable to respond or move. This was clearly an exceptionally low hypogly-caemic episode. Having no training and no understanding of what was happening, Mum first tried to make me eat some lollies but has vivid memories of me being extraordinarily strong and clamping my jaw shut. Next came a phone call to the hospital whose immediate response was to call 000. Unfortunately, by the time the ambulance arrived I had slid into a deep coma. To give credit where credit is due my life was saved by the fast action of both the emergency teams and physician who were able to administer glucose via an IV and restore the supply of glucose to my brain.

While I have no recollection of those two days, I do have rec-ollection of how I felt when I regained consciousness. Having no idea where I was or what had happened, what I do recall is once again being told off, as soon as I opened my eyes, for injecting insulin THEN having a shower before eating breakfast! Hmm, an offer of paracetamol for my extraordinary "hypo" headache would have been a particularly empathetic gesture. But I guess you need to ask an indi-vidual how they are feeling to determine how to help them.

Again, forty something years ago, there was no counselling for me, my family, and no real thought of what the physiological impact of such a significant event may be. Just the blame game ONCE again. The one thing it did cement was my determination not to ever return to the physician who had been overseeing my diabetes. Not because there may have been a mistake made and not even because I had

had a very memorable incident in my diabetes journey. But because it finally gave me a reason for me to refuse to continue attending a health professional whose idea of health care was based around blame and language I did not appreciate, child or not.

CHAPTER 3

Eggs in a Basket

The severe hypoglycaemic episode had more far-reaching consequences than one would anticipate. Sure, there are the obvious things. For years after my experience, I was unwilling to go to sleep at night unless my blood glucose level was above 10 mmol/L and sometimes even higher (maybe 15 mmol/L). While I do not have any recollection of the events leading up to the coma, I now had an overwhelming fear of going to sleep and not waking up.

I had learnt a couple of years back at diabetes camp, short bursts of above target glucose results caused no real harm except making me feel unwell. However, long periods above target cause complications. I also remember at diagnosis of my diabetes being told not to worry too much about the long-term complications because "these wouldn't occur for more than 20 years and by that time they will have found a cure". The obvious fix for feeling overwhelmed about nocturnal hypos was just to run my blood glucose levels above target all the time. Fixed. Oh, and I didn't need to worry about the long term since, like most other individuals, I had "it won't happen to me" belief. And, after all, if the health care team continued to accuse me of such things as eating when I really was not and sneaking food when I really, really was not, then I might as well do so! If you are going to be in trouble for something you did not do, I reasoned, I may as well do it and enjoy it! Again, the human "it won't happen to me" aspect of complications prevented me from ever really thinking about the future.

What I never had any real understanding or insight about was the impact of my diabetes on my family. This took years and came at a time when I least expected it. Having been to university and spent years working in the health industry, I had the opportunity to attend diabetes camp as an adult to help look after individuals in the same age group as when I had attended as a child. Interacting with these kids for three days, seeing the uncertainty of their parents as they handed the management of their children over to someone they have only just met, and performing numerous glucose levels in the middle of sleepless nights gave me an exceedingly small understanding of my parents' life. And how that severe hypoglycaemic episode must have rocked them to their very core. I now understand my Mum asking me what every SINGLE blood glucose reading was, every SINGLE day of every SINGLE week. And if I had injected my insulin, AND if I had eaten the right amounts of food. My adult self has perfect understanding of why this occurred and perfect patience. My teenage self, not so much! And hence the constant and consistent battles between my Mum and I. I wanted independence and would assert this by any means and at any cost. My Mum just wanted to know I was safe and well and okay. Never an easy solution and certainly a struggle that impacts families daily even today, despite enormous advances in technology and medicine.

Nonetheless we continued to manage as best we could as a family with amazing support from friends throughout my schooling until graduation and my move to Adelaide, some 600 plus kms away from my parents to begin University life.

It was at this time that my life changed considerably. Gone was the structured eating regimen. No regular lunch and dinner times like school anymore! This was uni! Great. How is that going to work for me? Luckily science, technology and medicine had "caught up" to some degree and we now had some newer insulin available. These were designed to fit around your schedule rather than you fitting around injecting and eating times. Ok, so instead of injecting twice a day and mixing my insulin and then eating regimented meals with regimented amounts of carbohydrates, I could now inject four times a day before each meal. That was the downside! One long-acting insulin to "feed" my cells glucose through out the day and night and give them energy, and three short acting injections to cover my meals. These short acting injections could be adjusted depending on what and how much I ate so I was not committed to eating the same amounts of food nor at the same time of the day. There was an upside! University started and so did my new diabetes management.

Despite this new era in my management, it was not until I had finished my degree, ironically in the health field, that I began to understand the poor relationship I had developed with food. Somewhere along the diagnosis and management curve of my diabetes, food was no longer enjoyable for me. Food had become my enemy. Despite attending my appointments with the dietitians as recommended and required, I was still unable to match the doses of short acting insulin to the amount of carbohydrates I consumed at meals to arrive at a satisfactory glucose level two hours after any one meal. Maybe one out of every twenty meals I would luck a satisfactory result. But do not ask me what I did and if I tried to repeat it with the same meal, I could never get that same result. Often, I would have a glucose level above target, which meant more insulin and more injections, but this could often result in more hypoglycaemic episodes in any one day and more calorie intake. This overall pattern led to weight gain. Not something any person wants but particularly hard for me as a young, impressionable female. Food became a numbers game, made up of complicated mathematical equations with no real benefit. My HbA1c really did not shift much. Yep, that magical number of 7 still eluded me. The irony (a very dear friend pointed out to me) that the unlucky number 13 was my glucose level at diagnosis and the lucky number 7 (with respect to HbA1c) remained so elusive to me. From my perspective all that was happening was weight gain from eating lollies when I continued to have hypos. Even participating in regular physical activity did not seem to help because I would often need to consume enormous amounts of calories before and after to prevent and treat hypos. Which really defeated the purpose of treadmills and gyms and everything else I continued to try and continued to invest time in.

I do remember becoming significantly overwhelmed with everything in about my second year of university. It took time (and courage) to go to my then specialist I was seeing while at university and try to discuss how I felt. Individuals with chronic health conditions, including diabetes, are twice as likely to experience mental health difficulties, including depression. This however is still not widely recognised and was certainly not well understood forty years ago. When I stumbled through my questions about how others feel and cope with diabetes, hypos, the worry of complications, weight and the stress of it all, the specialist started bumbling on about eggs in a basket! People with diabetes have more eggs to juggle and that's why they find sometimes they are more tired! No help with how I was feeling at all! Not that I expected any solutions because there aren't any really are there? But something better than eggs surely? Perhaps it was just the timing because we now have much better recognition and referral pathways and I would hope if this same situation presented itself, I would have much better hope of being referred to someone I could talk to about how I felt and have more of an opportunity to explore what I was currently dealing with.

Even today despite education and positive reinforcement and promotion, mental health has a stigma attached. It has taken several years and a team of health care professionals I not only love but have enormous respect for, that I have finally learnt where it fits in the bigger scheme of things. While studying one of my post graduate diplomas it became apparent that in almost every aspect of my life, I am very proactive. My A type personality deals best if I can categorise and then go about solving whatever comes my way. Diabetes makes me compromise on proactivity forcing me to be reactive more times a day than I would like, and this annoys me. Not the compromise itself but the fact I have inner conflict. Recognising this does not mean it is automatically resolved! However, it does allow certain clarification and the ability to accept that I may require extra help along the way. It certainly does not make me weaker nor that any one thing has got "the better" of me. Rather, I believe I have gained insight to help manage my diabetes on a much higher level.

I do however wish this insight and the health care team I now have could have occurred at a much earlier period of my diabetes journey. Having been sent away after the egg and basket "talk" I felt unable to revisit this subject for many years. Through my twenties and early thirties what then ensued was the yo-yoing that is often seen with many individuals with inner conflict. I struggled with hypos, weight gain, relationship break downs and HbA1c levels that I was forever reprimanded for. For a period, I stopped going to see all health professionals because I did not see the point of exposing myself to the constant barrage of reprimand. I also unfortunately developed an eating disorder. Having studied diabetes and worked out above target glucose levels caused frequent urination, I was able to calculate that if I lowered or even omitted insulin doses, I could lose weight. Years later I have learnt I am not alone with this and it is quite common. In fact, according to Diabetes Victoria, eating disorders are a significant health issue for people with diabetes, especially as a teenager. Although I was a little older than this, I had not escaped the fact that I had a serious detrimental relationship with food, because it had, along with my multiple daily injections and physical activity, became my major focus. The problem with what Diabetes Victoria terms "insulin-purging" (reducing or omitting insulin to "purge" calories) is it can cause significant long-term health consequences. Glucose is such a large molecule and irritates all the body including the nerves in the feet and hands causing neuropathy. Above target glucose levels over long periods of time can also cause damage to the eyes, heart, kidneys, and stomach to name a few.

However once again I was in the zone of "it won't happen to me". No amount of scare tactics will work long term on an individual. Telling me I might have eye, kidney, feet, or heart issues "later" in life is really not relevant when I am in the present struggling with self esteem issues and worrying if I am going to wake up in the morning because of a hypoglycaemic episode overnight!

CHAPTER 4

The 9/11

September 11, 2001 is a date that will be etched into the minds of most of the population of the world for all the wrong reasons. Waking up to horrific images of planes flying into the Twin Towers is something that will forever be firmly cemented in my mind. I am unable to comprehend what the victims and their families endured.

This date has a double significance for me. It was on this day I was diagnosed with vision threatening diabetes related retinopathy.

I had decided earlier in 2001 to have Lasik eye surgery to correct my short sightedness so I did not have to wear glasses or contact lenses. It is a reasonably easy procedure using a laser to correct short, or far, sightedness. I was incredibly happy with my decision, and results, and enjoyed no glasses or contacts for about six months before I started to notice a blurring around road signs and that my vision was just not as sharp as it had been when the operation was first performed.

Booked on this day for an appointment with the surgeon who had performed the Lasik surgery, I expected him to tell me that the slight change in my vision was completely normal and I needed to possibly return to have some minor alterations. Nope! Unfortunately, what he found was bleeding behind both my retinas! This condition was unrelated to the Lasik surgery but stemmed from years of stubbornly high blood glucose levels as a child and later as a young adult struggling to accept my condition and forgive my imperfections.

The retina is positioned in the back of the eye and acts like a lens in a camera. When images come into the eye and are focused on the retina, it converts them to signals that sends these via the optical nerve to the brain so we can make decisions about what we see. The retina has a rich blood supply and above target glucose levels can damage these exceedingly small vessels over time. Untreated retinopathy can cause significant visual loss and blindness.

So it was on September 11th 2001 I was given the news that I had vision threatening retinopathy and three days later on 14th September, I had my first laser treatment to try to prevent me going blind.

Proliferative retinopathy caused by diabetes is quite interesting, and certainly much more fascinating if it is not happening to you! During the early stages of retinopathy, above glucose levels damage the tiny blood vessels in the retina. Usually, individuals do not notice any change in their vision at this point, which is exactly what happened to me. I did not notice any difference in my vision at all. As the retinopathy progresses, new fragile blood vessels start to grow to replace the damaged ones. It is these new vessels that can bleed, leak, cloud vision and eventually destroy the retina. The idea behind scattered laser treatment is to destroy the abnormal blood vessels before they can destroy the eye. This treatment however does burn the retina and while it does reduce the vision lost through retinopathy, does itself cause visual loss, not correctable by any glasses or contact lens.

And despite my specialist telling me there would be little pain, I can honestly tell you there is nothing I have EVER experienced that has come close to the pain from the numerous laser treatments I then endured every two weeks for two years after that first time. Even pain numbing injections into the eye as a block to help stop me feeling the laser burning my eye wore off long before they were supposed to, leaving me with what I can only described as an ice cream headache multiplied by a billion! Fortunately, I am blessed with the most supportive, amazing, empathetic friend who also happens to be the most supportive, amazing, empathetic nurse. Not only did she accompany to almost each and every one of these torturous appointments and distract me when I wanted to run screaming from the surgery and NEVER come back, she made me laugh at her stupid jokes, and nursed me with incredible compassion after the operations when I was unable to lift my head due to pain.

And again, the irony of the laser was the more I had to save my eyesight, the more eyesight I lost.

While I do not believe being diagnosed with retinopathy was a good event in my life, it certainly made me realise I was taking my health for granted and if I did not like the status quo, then the only one who could change things was me! Welcome back from your diabetes holiday! As an A type personality, it was time to take charge.

Still under the same specialist I had been after my severe hypoglycaemic episode and I was at university, I wanted to explore the option of insulin pump therapy and whether it would be possible to use this as a treatment option for my diabetes. I do not actually recall where I first came across information about insulin pumps, but I do remember reading that they could help those individuals that found it difficult to manage above target glucose levels and those who have widely fluctuating results. Ready to have a conversation, I asked about the new technology. Like the eggs and the basket conversation, although with much more abruptness, I was told simply, insulin pump therapy was "not suitable" for me and was, "in fact, far too dangerous".

Although in 2001, the pumps did not have any of the "smart" features currently available today (such as custom alarms, bolus calculators and food databases), they were certainly small devices with technology I wanted to explore as a way of managing my diabetes.

It was at this point I decided once again I needed to change specialists. Not because the specialist did not want to change me over to an insulin pump but simply because he was not prepared to allow a discussion. After all, who has the diabetes? Who lives with it day in, day out? Yes, he had the qualifications and expertise, but I wanted to have some input in my health condition. Health care professionals have a say in my diabetes less than 1% of the time and I have to manage it the other 99%. By now I was working as a health professional and consistently recommended that clients use only reputable internet sites. Yet here I was, despite the perils of search engines, searching the Internet for an endocrinologist who specialised in pump therapy. As luck would have it the search engine at the time happened across an endocrinologist I am often known to refer to as "God" although better probably described as one of the most knowledgeable, empathetic, understanding health professionals I am lucky to have in my team.

When meeting with him at my first appointment to discuss insulin pump therapy, he asked me why I wanted an insulin pump. Keep in mind this was back in 2001 when the pump consumables (the tubing that attaches the person to the pump) were not funded by the government. So yes, they were expensive. However, my understanding (and back then I had extraordinarily little understanding of pumps) was that they could manage glucose levels much better than multiple daily injections.

While rudimentary years ago, pumps allow an extra amount of short acting insulin two hours after food (without the need for another injection) so an individual does not remain above target for longer than necessary. Even the most dedicated individual on multiple injections does not usually have another injection after a meal. They usually just wait for the next meal to correct above target glucose levels. They also allow for long-acting insulin to be removed because you are connected to the pump which only uses short acting insulin, although you can disconnect for up to 2 hours at a time. The pump takes over the job of the long-acting insulin (called the basal rate), releasing a small amount automatically. The basal rate can be changed every half to one hour, making the Dawn Phenomenon so much easier to deal with. And the relationship with food becomes much more balanced and closer to normality. Hypoglycaemia is also much easier to treat on an insulin pump due to the fact there is only the short acting insulin to think about when treating the low blood glucose result.

Having been diagnosed with retinopathy not two months before sourcing a new endocrinologist, I was once again doing my utmost to reduce my blood glucose levels to within target. This meant monitoring up to twenty times a day, including in the middle of the night, and sometimes having up to twelve injections a day. It also meant some overly concerning hypos again. So when I explained what had been happening, my new endocrinologist's comment was that I had some pretty good reasons for wanting to try pump therapy. He was prepared to have a conversation about it, thought all seemed reasonable and better yet, was happy to move forward.

December 2001, I started insulin pump therapy. Was it hard work for the first three months? Absolutely! I remember going to sleep in hospital on the first night of the changeover (years ago when insulin pump therapy was started for the first time there was a 48-hour admission to hospital to learn how the pump works) with my insulin pump on my chest. Given that this "machine" was going to be responsible for keeping me alive, I wanted to make damn sure it was always working!

So why do I believe insulin pump therapy is of benefit for my diabetes? There are several reasons for this. One of the most significant for me is the removal of long-acting insulin. Insulin pumps only use ultra short acting insulin, which is why you are connected to them (via tubing) most of the day. The general rule of thumb is that you can disconnect for a maximum of two hours, however once again my diabetes tends to not follow the usual patterns and I am simply not able to disconnect for any more than about 15 minutes. The pump automatically gives a small amount of insulin every couple of minutes (called a basal rate) which takes over the job of the long-acting insulin. In fact, it has been widely recognised that pump therapy is the closest we have to delivering insulin similar to that which is delivered by a pancreas. Without a doubt removing long-acting insulin made me instantly feel better. Less sluggish and much more alert if I could describe it that way.

I was also able to immediately manage my Dawn Phenomenon because I could adjust my basal rate at night for just a couple of hours when this was occurring. I also spent a month after starting pump therapy eating vegetables with my meals and I really didn't even enjoy the taste of vegetables. Do you know why? Because I could! Hypoglycaemia was also so much easier for me to treat and because I was able to reduce the amount of insulin I was giving with each of my meals and snacks (called a bolus), I had less hypos. I have a saying "what goes in my mouth, goes in my pump". Any form of carbohydrate, no matter what it is I put the amount in my insulin pump and the pump converts the grams of carbohydrate and any refined sugar to units of insulin. The pump is also able to give much smaller amounts of insulin compared to needles or an insulin pen allowing for a finer dosing schedule. Once again, better management for me and my diabetes. While insulin pumps years ago were considerably basic, I still had much more confidence in managing my diabetes this way than I had previously. The one hindrance was, and still is, the cost. Diabetes is an awfully expensive health condition and while there is some compensation under Medicare and the NDSS (National Diabetes Service Scheme) the pump consumables were not covered in 2001. This meant the syringe that holds the insulin in the pump, the tubing that connected me to the pump and the needle that I inserted every three to four days under my skin were not funded by the government or private health insurance and were very costly at the time. Worth it? Absolutely! The benefits of insulin therapy far outweighed the disadvantages.

Interestingly, about three months after spending two nights in hospital on a steep learning curve changing my diabetes management it suddenly hit me I still had diabetes! And retinopathy. I know that sounds ridiculous, but I had spent 18 years of my life having fought with above target glucose levels no matter what I did or how hard I worked. Then suddenly insulin pump therapy had changed that! Hard work now meant I was rewarded with a HbA1c for the first time in target range. It was almost like finding a cure. So, three months after embracing pump therapy there was a realisation that I really did still have type 1. Oh, and complications. Bugger.

There are however benefits of insulin pump therapy that have nothing to do with diabetes or health! As mentioned previously every visit to my ophthalmologist I was accompanied by my dear friend who would inevitably make me laugh. She too has type 1 diabetes and chooses insulin pump therapy to manage this. We met when we were admitted to hospital to learn about these devices that were going to be attached to our bodies.

Not only has she been my confidante, my nurse, my travel companion, my driver, my ride partner, and my friend, she has been like a sister to me.

Having travelled through two years of what I will only describe as laser hell, I had survived and come out the other side. Fortunately, despite losing some eyesight from the laser itself, my retinopathy was stable and has remained that way for quite a few years. I have my eye specialist to thank for that! We often joke, at my yearly check, about having some laser for old time's sake. I am sure you can guess what answer I am quick to reply with.

To be fair, it's important to understand insulin pumps are not without their disadvantages. There is no long-acting insulin on board, something I enjoyed immediately because as previously stated it made me feel better. However, when something goes wrong it can go wrong very, very quickly. The lines that deliver the insulin can get blockages and I am always vigilant about my set changes. In fact, I was excited when first choosing pump therapy because I thought I would be able to downsize my handbag. Wrong! I now carry at least one of everything with me every where I go. This includes a battery, insulin cartridge, pump tubing, and pump syringe. Going through an airport is a nightmare. However, over the years I have learnt to problem solve almost every scenario that has happened. One of these is that the cannulas which deliver insulin under the skin kept bending which stopped the flow of insulin, causing prolonged and frequent elevated glucose results. The solution? Stainless steel needles sitting under the skin rather than Teflon. Sounds uncomfortable but I find them much more reliable, and my body appears to react much less to them.

However, me being me, insulin pump therapy did not solve all my diabetes management issues. Despite my HbA1c finally hitting target, I still had widely fluctuating glucose levels. At any given point of the day, I had glucose levels well above or well below target.

So, while I had finally managed to hit one of the bullseyes (HbA1c now well within the target range), diabetes stability still eluded me. This became particularly concerning as the lower my HbA1c became, the more hypoglycaemic episodes crept in. And so became my dilemma that I had been faced with on more than one occasion. Higher HbA1c and run the risk of more complications especially with my eyes, or lower HbA1c and have very, very scary hypos, even with an insulin pump.

CHAPTER 5

Insulin Pump "Connections"

As I look back through many of the experiences in my life, I have come to the realisation that although it took some time to develop into the person I am today, I always had the potential because of my incredible parents. This goes further than my diabetes; they gave me permission to stand up for what was right, not only for others but also for myself. As a result, I had found a supportive endocrinologist who understood that managing a chronic health condition like diabetes was hard work, and that I was a person and not just a number or a health state. I also, for one of the first times in my life, connected with others with type 1 diabetes; maybe because I was ready to accept my condition, or maybe it was just because it was the right time.

I finally felt comfortable to tell my health professionals what I needed and what I wanted. And so, from this defining moment I have surrounded myself with only health professionals that do not blame, do not "tell" me what to do and ALWAYS treat with the respect that I deserve as a PERSON and not a HEALTH CONDITION.

Insulin pump therapy has improved my quality of life beyond anything I am ever able to describe on a quality-of-life survey. How do you explain the difference in the relationship with food you have, how you feel about your body and body image, the fear of nocturnal hypoglycaemia, and the constant and consistent battling for the unachievable numbers? I am happy to admit there were days I really did not want to be connected to a "machine". While they were few and far between, when I felt like this, disconnecting, and going for a brisk walk for a short period of time worked for me. Having nothing attached helped my mindset and the brisk walk helped with glucose levels for the time without insulin. While the rule of thumb with insulin pump therapy is that an individual can be disconnected to anywhere up to two hours, this "rule" of course, did not work well for my body. Even now the maximum I can disconnect from my pump before the lack of insulin begins to influence my blood glucose levels is approximately 15 minutes. Therefore, when I do occasionally disconnect, I offset any "spikes" in glucose levels with some physical activity.

What also helped me through all the minefield of ups and downs was peer support. I have made so many special and lifelong friends through having diabetes and I have been very fortunate in so many ways to have such a beautiful, caring network as close as my family. I continue to do this no matter how long I have diabetes. This very book was edited by a beautiful lady I have much respect for and hold dear to my heart. Alex, who also connected to a pump in 2001 was, and still is, one of many who provide great support; talking about issues that arise can never be underrated.

I also connected with an organisation known as JDRF (Juvenile Diabetes Research Foundation).

While we no longer call type 1 "juvenile diabetes", JDRF is still recognised around the world by this name, although they support all people with type 1 diabetes, no matter what their age. JDRF's mission is to accelerate life-changing breakthroughs to cure, prevent and treat type 1 diabetes and its long-term health consequences.

Having already connected with Alex, she convinced me we needed to ride a bike through the undulating (this is a word that describes hills when you do not actually want to use the word HILL) landscape of the beautiful Barossa Valley to raise funds for JDRF. And beautiful it is, except when you have seen it on a bicycle 11 times. Do not get me wrong, the scenery doesn't change, just my appreciation of it really! I hate cycling, I hate cycling with a passion. Yet I have turned up in January year after year since the first ride to continue fundraising for JDRF but also for the peer support.

Some individuals are there because JDRF run an amazing event and support the riders. I have often heard from cyclists that have participated in many cycling events, that the JDRF Ride to Cure is one of the best organised events, a credit to everyone involved year after year. Others, like me, have an emotional and personal connection to type 1 diabetes. I probably have mentioned I do not enjoy cycling, right? So, to continue to turn up year after year gives you some indication of the connection I feel with others and how powerful peer support can be. Since The Ride commencement, I have maintained a strong connection with JDRF for all events: Walk to Cure, Ride to Cure, Jump to Cure, Gala ball, and jelly baby campaign. I have also made some amazing lifelong friends through the organisation who have, and continue to be, enormous support along my journey with my life experiences and my diabetes.

Finding the right support has been essential to maintaining a healthy relationship with my diabetes and at that stage in my life I had finally found what I needed.

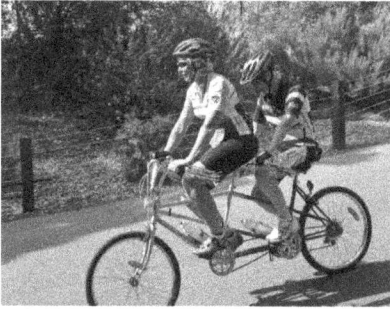

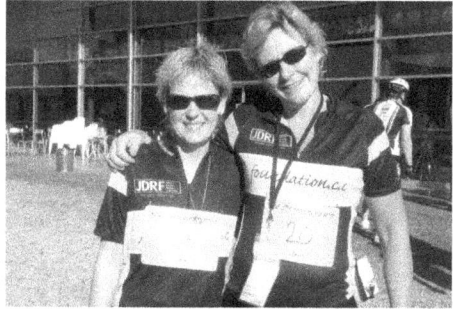

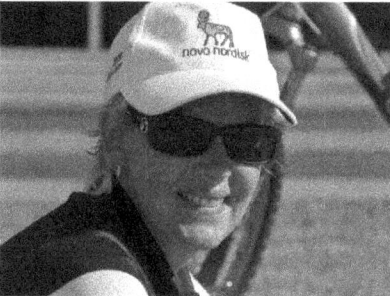

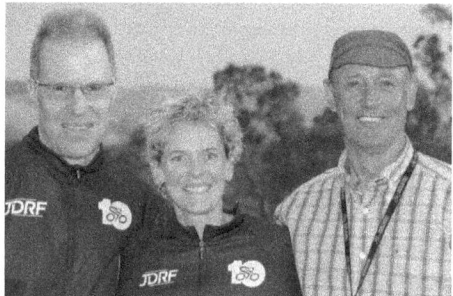

My dear friend Alex and I "mixing it up a bit" on the 2010 and 2011 Ride to Cure Diabetes (top left). Smiles all round as I finished the Ride to Cure, 2010 (top right). Friends and me at Ride to Cure 2012 (bottom).

While the pump allowed me to participate in the Ride to Cure it, however, did not fix everything. Just because my HbA1c, was now hitting target for the first time in my life, it did not mean my widely fluctuating glucose levels or my daily (or more) hypoglycaemic episodes were fixed. In fact, my low glucose levels got lower (because my glucose levels overall had reduced). To fix these lows, I would have to eat significantly more food, causing rebound above target glucose levels. This in turn meant correction insulin doses and a constant yo-yo effect. Despite amazing support from my health care team, here came diabetes burn out again. This time it was made worse by a couple of health consequences: retinopathy, although stable, and a new health outcome from long term diabetes, hypoglycaemic unawareness.

Affecting less than 1% of individuals with diabetes, hypoglycae-mic unawareness means I have the inability to determine when my blood glucose levels are dropping below target (under 4 mmol/L). If left untreated due to no symptoms, then I am in real danger of lapsing into a coma. The opposite, of course is true. I have no ability to determine if my blood glucose levels are above target. At the time the only way to know what my glucose result was at any given time was to monitor. Lots. Day and night. Monitoring at night is a dou-ble-edged sword. If I did not wake up and perform a finger stick, then I might drop dangerously low. However, setting alarms every night and breaking my sleep pattern started to wear me out quickly - I am sure I don't have to explain that to any parents of newborns or small infants. At some point this fatigue causes the potential to sleep through a hypoglycaemic episode despite having alarms set. Remember this was all before continuous glucose monitoring was available.

Having such widely fluctuating glucose levels also played havoc in many other areas of my life. I found it extremely difficult to deal with incredible swings in my moods. Although amazingly comfortable with my health care team, mental health has such a stigma. The Australian Institute of Health and Welfare recognizes that "Australians with dia-betes are significantly more likely than other Australians to have poor mental health and well being." It took a long time to recognise it was okay to admit that I was not coping. Whether that was the impact of swinging glucose levels or the impact of realising I was living with a chronic condition, is probably something that will never be able to be separated. So, despite my bad experience years ago with the "egg and basket" talk that will remain with me forever, I was now prepared to revisit the idea with a team I felt comfortable talking to.

Widely fluctuating glucose levels also played havoc with my eye-sight. Having lost a significant amount of vision ironically to save my sight, the swings between above and below target glucose results affected my ability to see clearly. That, coupled with the risk of hypoglycaemia, made me realise it was time to surrender my driver's licence. I was no longer safe to myself or others and felt this was the most responsible thing to do. But wow what an impact on my life. It meant selling the house I was living in and moving closer to Adelaide so that I was able to access better resources. I am very thankful that I worked for an amazingly understanding group of health professionals who, at the time, immediately located my workplace closer to my home so that I was less dependent on public transport. The irony however was I spent most of my time walking, or (despite my original dislike!) cycling, everywhere. Physical activity is something I have always enjoyed and embraced as a management tool for my diabetes, among other benefits. However sometimes after, or during, exercise I would have a hypoglycaemic episode, despite turning my basal rate on my pump down (that is, reducing the basal rate temporarily), and eating before, during and after. At other times, my glucose levels would be well above target (due to the "feel good" hormones released during said exercise) and would stay this way for up to twelve hours after finishing the activity. There was never any rhyme or reason and never a trend. Trying to plan for the effects of physical activity I was now participating in every day became incredibly challenging. My increase in activity also made my hypos more pronounced, especially at night, despite adjusting insulin doses and basal rates many times.

Having tried every avenue and with me now being unable to detect any drop in blood glucose levels, my endocrinologist spoke to me about a new procedure to treat type 1 diabetes being undertaken at Westmead Hospital in Sydney known as "islet cell transplantation".

CHAPTER 6

What is an Islet?

What the average person, often even one with diabetes, does not understand is that individuals with type 1 diabetes have a working pancreas. It is estimated an adult has approximately one million islets of Langerhans (the cells that produce insulin) which make up just 1-2% of the pancreas. These cells are what my body's immune system attacked and destroyed when I was young. It makes sense therefore rather than transplanting the whole pancreas to just transplant the islet cells. This means smaller doses of immune suppression therapy are needed to prevent the body's immune system causing rejection and therefore there are fewer short- and long-term side effects from the immune suppressant medicine.

While doing a little research for this book, I learnt that islet transplantation is not a new concept. Apparently, an English surgeon by the name of Charles Pybus (1882-1975) attempted to cure type 1 diabetes by grafting pancreatic tissue. This method was described in a diabetes journal in 1967. However, it was not until the refinement of anti-rejection medicines (first published in the England Journal of Medicine I July 2000) that islet grafting really became popular as a treatment option for hypoglycaemic unawareness. These medicines allowed corticosteroids to be removed from the regimen but still allowed viability of the transplanted cells. ((While corticosteroids protect islet cells from rejection from the body's immune system, they also increase insulin resistance long term. Ironically this makes the transplanted cells fatigue over time and can cause steroid induced diabetes).

Given few to no alternatives and the amazing swings in my every day glucose levels, my endocrinologist suggested I might like to consider this option. Australian trials had begun on six individuals with type 1 diabetes and had been undertaken at Westmead Hospital in Sydney as a joint exercise between the National Pancreas Transplant Unit and the Department of Endocrinology.

And so, began my "suitability determination". You name an "ologist" I reckon I have seen one for nearly every part of my body to make sure that I was a suitable candidate for islet cell transplantation.

Thanks to the amazing people who have agreed to be donors in the event of their death, islet cells can be removed from their pancreas for transplant. The process includes the use of special enzymes within a device called a Ricordi's Chamber.

Believe it or not, transplantation occurs not into the pancreas but into the liver. The liver can grow new blood vessels to supply nutrients to the donor cells and keep them viable (alive). To prevent rejection of a cellular mass that is not my own which my body's immune system will recognise as foreign, anti-rejection medicine must be taken every day. As with all medicines, these have side effects, including high cholesterol, high blood pressure, changes to kidney function (ironic with someone with diabetes as this is what we try to prevent in the first place!), as well as those issues causally related to having a lowered immune system, such as slow healing of wounds, and an increased risk of cancer.

Due to the fact that islet transplantation was still in trial phases, there had to be a consensus by all those concerned that I would have more to gain by going ahead than by remaining status quo. Because of the severity of my hypoglycaemic events, I was ready to move forward. Luckily, all of the medical team agreed.

And so began the next phase. First with a letter to the Westmead doctor involved in selecting possible candidates for islet transplantation, asking for consideration. Then came an actual meeting with the specialist who would make the final decision as to whether I would qualify! At Westmead! In Sydney! I do not remember much of that actual meeting except being totally overwhelmed by how extraordinarily large the hospital was and how many people were all sitting in waiting rooms everywhere.

At the time one of my girlfriends that I used to go to school with was living in Sydney and she came with me to the hospital. Having been sent to wait in one of the enormous waiting rooms, I remember waiting for an awfully long time before Kirstin took it upon herself to go and seek some information about why it was taking so long for my turn. Uh oh, as it turns out we had been sent to the wrong department and they had been paging me over at another department for over an hour. Racing over to meet the professor who was running the trial, I then had less than 15 minutes to explain to him why I felt I should be a candidate before having to race off to meet the team's endocrinologist, at her rooms. Normally she would see candidates at the hospital but given the mix up with the waiting rooms, she was unable to stay. These two meetings may have been the most important meetings of my life, with some answers to the most important questions and I was rushing all over a strange city on a time schedule (my flight home was that afternoon) because somewhere someone had read my letter incorrectly and sent me on a wild goose chase! At this point in time, I can honestly say I was not entirely sure I wanted to have a transplant at Westmead!! Nonetheless arriving at the endocrinologist's office and meeting her had a profoundly calming influence on me. She asked me some very simple questions about my diabetes and what treatments I had tried in the past, explained to me the team had received a very thorough referral letter from my treating endocrinologist and reassured me they would take my case into very serious deliberation.

The criteria at the time for selection into islet cell transplantation (apart from having type 1 diabetes) was severe hypoglycaemic unawareness and very few other complications. This was due to the side effects of the antirejection medicines. So, while the diagnosis of retinopathy had rocked my world, for all intents and purposes it was not anything too dramatic from a medical perspective. Oh sure, it was devastating and overwhelming and so life changing, but from a life saving perspective it does not inhibit the body taking care of itself. So, retinopathy was not an issue for undergoing islet cell transplantation. Any other complications like kidney problems, heart damage, liver issues or neuropathy could have ruled me out so although lucky is not a word I often used to describe myself when it comes to health, so far so good it would seem.

And so began the many, many, many scans, tests, and procedures to determine if I indeed was a candidate. Blood and urine checks to determine kidney function, which included too many 24-hour urine samples to count. There are probably not too many people that have stopped and considered what a 24-hour sample procedure consists of but if you think about why it is named that then it is quite self explanatory. It's simply urinating in a bottle for 24 hours then taking this to a collection laboratory to have bloods taken as close to the end of the 24-hour period as possible so that both the urine and blood can be sent away together. So much fun, especially when you get to do it on more than a few occasions! Then came ultrasounds and liver scans to make sure my liver was able to accept the transplanted donor cells. Nerve studies also showed no issues at all so all positive so far for moving forward with the transplant work up. Then a stress test of my heart where I had to walk/run on a treadmill while hooked up to a heart monitor. I felt comfortable with this test given I had recently had a full check over by a cardiologist and he had given me the all-clear to continue with this next step. It was here that things took a little unexpected turn. The doctor and nurse overseeing my jogging on the treadmill in the hospital asked me to stop the stress test halfway through despite me telling them I was feeling fine and happy to continue. The doctor told me the cardiac monitor had detected an "abnormality" and that a report would be sent to both the referring cardiologist and endocrinologist. I think his parting words were "try not to worry until you see them". Oh, ok easy enough, NOT!

A phone call from my endocrinologist telling me the stress test had revealed quite serious damage to my heart gave me even more reason for concern until, once again, things were put into perspective. Given I had just participated in and completed a Ride to Cure Diabetes, my endocrinologist did not believe there was much chance this new revelation had much merit. However, it had to be proven inaccurate to continue to meet islet transplantation criteria. Okay next on the list? A coronary angiogram to determine if any of my arteries or valves in my heart were blocked.

Well, that cannot be too hard right? Again, a reasonably straightforward procedure for someone without diabetes but this can carry extra risk for those with diabetes. A catheter was inserted through a small incision in the groin (as was the practice in those days) and threaded to the heart. Once in place, a dye was injected which was then viewed on X-rays as it moved through the heart. The dye was then eliminated through the kidneys and a plug placed at the groin to create a seal once the catheter was removed. Due to the kidneys already being under stress when you have diabetes, extra pressure to eliminate a dye can be detrimental and so it was decided that an overnight stay in hospital would be a good idea so that I could have some fluids via IV to protect my kidneys.

I have a very hazy recollection of the angiogram due to a light sedative was given. I do remember feeling very sore in the groin for weeks afterwards and having to carry an identification card about the plug in my leg for three months. All things considered, it really was a simple procedure, especially given the outcome showed, as suspected, no major blockages and, functionally my heart was sound and could stand the anti-rejection medicines. Another hurdle overcome.

Next was a psychiatrist to determine if my mental health could withstand the pressures of a transplant. Unfortunately, as is almost always the case when dealing with transplantation, it is not about whether an individual "wants" a transplant. When considering this option, it's because almost every other alternative has been exhausted. I honestly do not believe that when I began my journey back in 2005 I was any different to any other individual waiting for a transplant. Except for one difference: this was a trial, not an established procedure, and there was no guarantee of success. While extremely nervous, I do remember the psychiatrist making me feel amazingly comfortable and explaining to me I was just having a conversation with him. I also remember coming away from the meeting feeling quite calm.

And so, after another couple of trips back and forth to Sydney, I was finally through and being blood typed and matched and placed on the waiting list! Good and ready to go. However, what an incredibly long waiting list it was, and as we are probably all aware, still is. In that year (2006) in Australia 2000 individuals were waiting for an organ donation and there were only 202 multi-organ donations.

I had a profound sense of hope when I finally made it to the list. No matter how hard my day with swinging glucose levels and no matter how low my hypoglycaemic episodes got, hope is an immensely powerful force that can change an individual's perspective on so many situations. Not even a severe hypo incident (I can distinctly remember dropping my glass lolly jar, continuing to sit in the middle of the glass and eat glass plus lollies, then laying down and sleeping in the middle of broken glass) could stop me feeling like I could finally move forward. Needless to say, no more glass lolly jars for me!

Waiting was incredibly hard however and amazingly stressful. It is something that I believe is totally underestimated. There are unwritten conditions that go with the expectation of transplantation, which I took very seriously, as I have no doubt every individual would in circumstances similar to me. This meant no alcohol, especially on occasions such as Easter, Christmas, and public holidays when there is a higher percentage of road fatalities. As morbid as it sounds, donations must come from somewhere and this is the reality of those waiting for a call. So each and every time my mobile rang, especially with a number I did not recognise or a blocked number (hospitals block outgoing calls) I had the overwhelming sense of both excitement and anticipation. And the phone therefore had to stay attached 24 hours a day, 7 days a week, always fully charged, never left at home, never left on silent, and never anywhere that did not have range! And no going further than about an hour from Adelaide airport.

Oh, and the other BIG kicker was that I had to lose some weight and fast. Insulin is calculated by a weight ratio. If the average healthy person has approximately one million islet cells then the lighter a person is, the less number of islets needed for transplantation. The Westmead team wanted me under 60 kg before transplantation so that the first lot of transplanted cells would not be put under too much insulin per kg pressure.

This may sound relatively easy, but everyone knows losing weight is hard at the best of times. Adding extra calories in the form of pure refined sugar every time I had a hypoglycaemic event made it that much harder. However, I was determined to do everything that was asked to ensure the success of the procedure. Jenny Craig here we come!

Having had my endocrinologist sign the form that stated I was able to participate in a weight loss program (one of the interesting facts about having diabetes, is the variety of things you are not able to do without a doctor's "say so") I began my strict eating regimen. No deviations except when I hypoed. And I joined a gym and hated every single minute!

As previously stated, the irony of physical activity is that usually it causes blood glucose levels to drop. However sometimes it can cause blood glucose levels to increase. This is because physical activity causes the release of "feel good" hormones which can compete with insulin's action and prevent it from working properly.

So sometimes when I went to the gym or took my dogs for a walk, I would be above target, sometimes hypoing but very rarely would I actually ever finish exercising and be right where I wanted to be, blood glucose wise. Frustrating from a glucose level and a weight perspective.

And then I found Bikram Yoga.

CHAPTER 7

Bikram

It is not my intention to convert anyone to Bikram yoga or even to regular yoga, but rather to simply share my experience.

Yoga is form of spiritual, mental, and physical routines that originated in India and was later introduced to western society in the late 19th century. One of the most popular forms of yoga is Hatha Yoga which places an emphasis on physical exercises to conquer the body, with a focus on diet and processes to aid in purification. Hatha Yoga benefits are like all other yogas: the physical postures (called asanas) develop body flexibility, relaxation, strength and personal concentration, along with breathing exercises (pranayamas), which help with meditation and spiritual development.

There is some literature describing the benefits of yoga. While there were 4450 reported injuries from all forms of yoga in the USA in 2006, there is growing evidence that yoga can be beneficial in diabetes, high blood pressure, asthma, chronic pain and heart disease. Those that practise regularly describe a decrease in alcohol consumption, better quality of sleep, lower levels of depression and anxiety, improved immune function, lower levels of stress, weight loss, improved strength, flexibility and circulation and reduced need for some medicines. There is also the advantage of an increased feeling of wellbeing and physical heath.

Bikram yoga is a form of Hatha yoga, developed by Bikram Choudhury who claims to have begun practising at age four. According to a 2013 study, after practicing Bikram yoga three times a week for eight weeks, healthy young adults noticed a reduction in body fat and an increase in flexibility and strength. While Bikram makes many other health claims for his 26 postures, there have been no medical studies to support his statements.

The Bikram method of Hatha Yoga is a series of 26 stretching and strengthening postures (asanas) with 2 breathing exercises performed at 40 degrees (Celsius). The series is scientifically designed to provide 100 percent total body workout from bones to skin, fingers to toes. By the end of the 90-minute workout, the claim is the yoga will have worked muscles, tendons, joints, and ligaments as well as internal organs and glands

There are also lots of reasons for yoga in 40 degrees! The heat speeds up the breakdown of glucose and fatty acids. Yoga has been shown to reduce stress and mange hyperglycaemia and increase uptake of glucose into the muscles. It has also been shown to enhance weight loss. What did I have to lose?

My good friend Alex always supportive of everything thing I did, could see I was really struggling with going to the gym. While my strict dieting with Jenny Craig was helping with some weight loss, I was finding it difficult to maintain the calorie restriction due to the number of hypos I was having. Alex had been going to Bikram for some weeks and had seen benefit in weight and diabetes management. She had been talking about it with me (one might use the word nag but I would NEVER!) and so on one of my days off work Alex took me to my first class!

My early recollection of my first Bikram class and the heat, my sweat and the sweat of all the other participants is not pleasant. Really? 90 minutes of this?????

Whether there is supporting evidence or studies that show it can help diabetes, or any other chronic condition has no real relevance to me. What is important is how it makes me feel and how it influences both the fluctuations in my glucose levels and my glucose levels themselves.

And so began my journey with Bikram yoga as a form of physical activity many years ago. What I have discovered over the years is it is so much more than just a physical work out for me. It is everything that is described in the benefits of yoga. While helping me lose and maintain the weight that was required by the transplant team (both in the short and long term), it has also taught me about meditation and emotional stability which has been of extreme value to my overall well-being in demanding times.

Some days I love it, some days I hate it. But even when I hate it, I love the feeling it gives me when I finish a class. I estimate it reduces one third of the dose of insulin I need each day and keeps my blood glucose levels extremely stable during the actual exercise itself, something no other form of exercise has been able to do for me. Does that mean I never hypo during class? Absolutely not!!! In fact, I am often having a snack while trying to do poses, although I do not recommend lollies and backward bends together!! My lolly pack, glucose tubes, blood glucose meter and soft drink that sit beside my yoga mat would put some picnics to shame.

And explaining to new yoga teachers what type 1 diabetes is, what my insulin pump is, why I may need to eat and why my pump sometimes beeps when the class is silent can be challenging. In fact, one teacher, albeit well meaning, told me Bikram would "cure" my diabetes and gave me a book to read. Yes, it was all about an individual who lost lots of weight having been diagnosed with type 2 diabetes and reduced his medicine. While remarkably interesting and entertaining reading, most people are unaware that type 1 and type 2 diabetes are such different health states! However, yoga (or any exercise or physical activity for that matter) makes people more insulin sensitive. Hence the reduced amount of insulin doses for me and much less medicine for the individual person with type 2 diabetes. Has practicing yoga cured my diabetes? Of course not! Has it helped? Absolutely! Which is why I keep going.

In fact, so dedicated to ensuring that I continue to practice yoga two to three times a week most weeks, I have been known to rearrange my week and holidays around yoga. That is the commitment I have to my physical and mental well-being. In fact, my idea of a holiday now encompasses yoga, or better yet, is a yoga retreat. I have been fortunate enough to have been on two Bikram yoga retreats, one in Koh Samui in 2014 and another one in Bali in 2015.

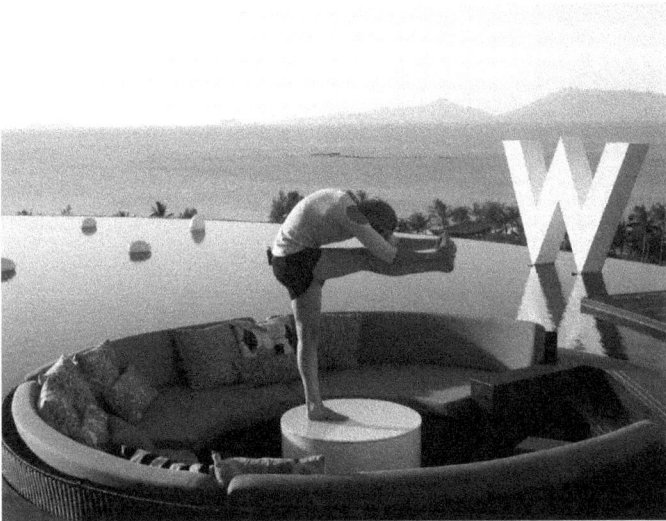

Standing Head to Knee Pose (Dandāyamana) in Koh Samui

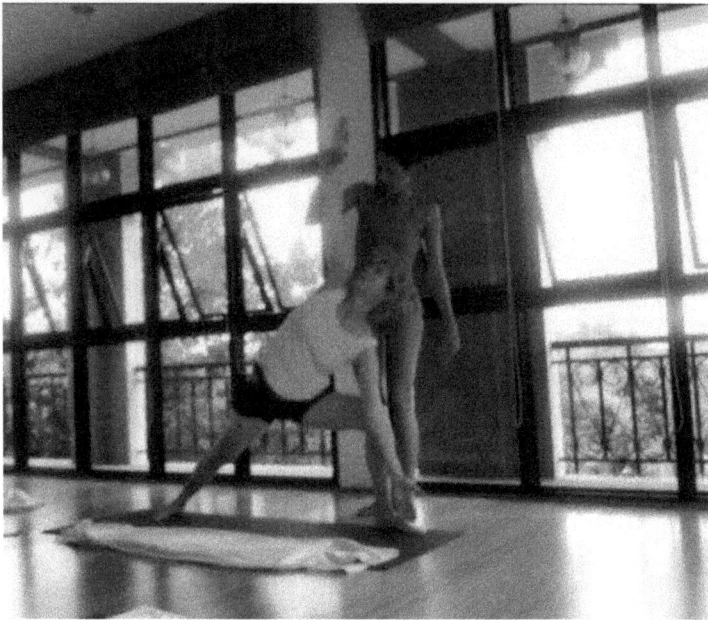

Fixed Firm Pose (Suptavajrāsana)

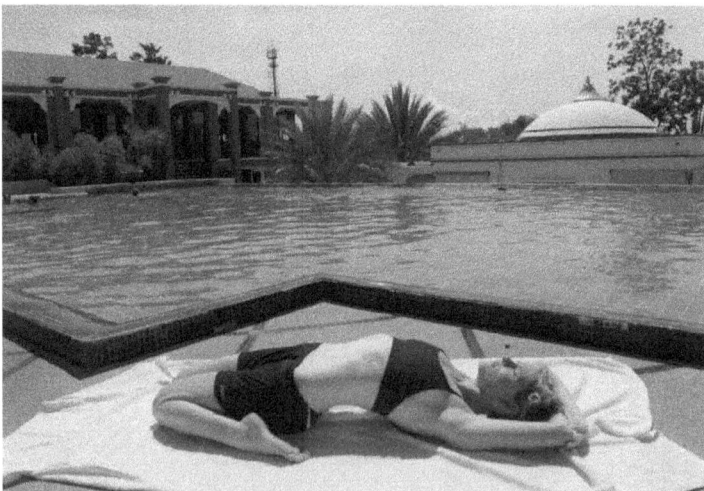

Triangle (Trikonāsaṇa) Pose

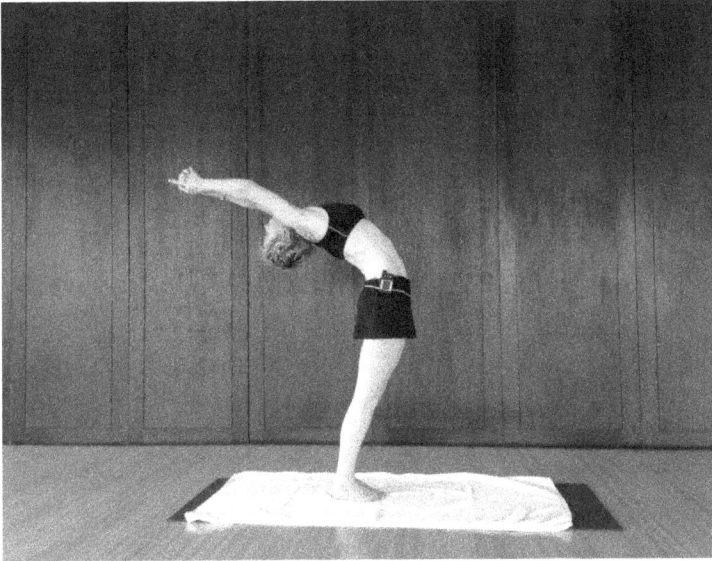

Back Bend with insulin pump on hip.
This photo was not set up! (Ardhacandrāsana)

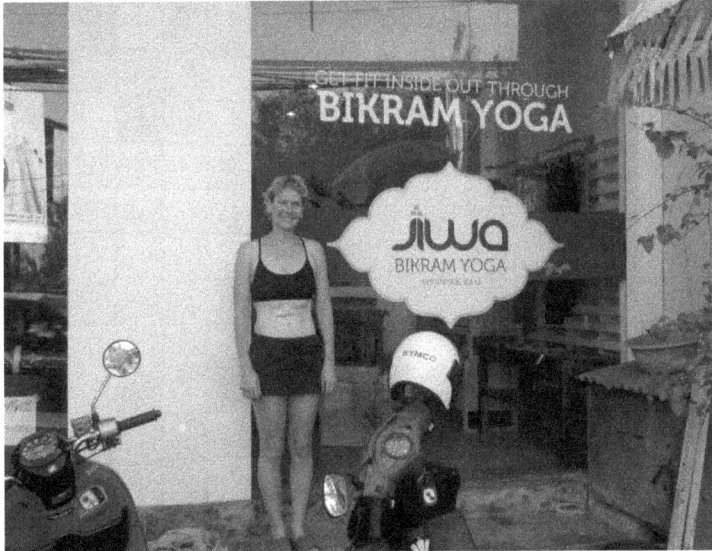

Bali 2015

Possibly more importantly it helped with my weight and body image, and stress levels, and acceptance of myself and others. There are over 100 schools of yoga including Hatha yoga, Raja (royal) yoga, Bikram yoga and Jnana (path of knowledge) yoga. However, despite different practices, the main purpose of yoga is to achieve clarity of mind and contentment. Physical activity plays an important role in the treatment of diabetes, no matter what type an individual has. Finding an activity that I loved doing was just as important as actually doing that activity because then it was maintainable long term. The fact that it had the other benefits stabilising my glucose levels and calming my mind was an extra bonus. This was especially important given the extra stress waiting for a call and the pressure of constantly watching calories.

And so, I settled into a routine of two to three yoga classes a week, Jenny Craig food and a waiting game.

CHAPTER 8

Doritos

Wednesday May 30th, 2007, started much like any other day. My Mum and Dad had been staying for a couple of days but were leaving that morning to drive back to Port Lincoln where they still lived. To save me having to walk to work they were going to drop me off there as they left. Sitting chatting just after breakfast, my phone rang.

The Westmead transplant coordinator identified himself on the other end of the phone and although I do not remember his exact words, I do remember him asking me if I had had a nice weekend. He then told me he had quite a busy one because he had spent it isolating islet cells from a donor and he just wanted to know if maybe I wanted to come on over and accept them. While I know that's what he does for a job, I was quite shocked by how calm he sounded! He told me he would ring me back with flights for the afternoon but that I should pack a bag! How panicked I became having to run around packing for at least one month (for this was the time I knew I would have to stay in Sydney recovering) and organise someone to cover me at work for the day and the following time that I would be away. Oh, and then get to the airport in time for the impending flight.

While I was running around the house Mum and Dad as always were there to support and help me in any way they could. Having always lived in the country and being the only one who held a licence until Damien and I were old enough this day is the only time I ever remember Dad offering to drive me to Adelaide! Dad was uncomfortable to drive in the BIG city (if I could even describe Adelaide as this). And so once again having contacted Alex to see me off at the airport Mum and Dad helped load my suitcase in the car and drop me at Alex's (who would later take me to the airport) while my parents headed home (although not without me promising I would keep them updated as much as possible)!

By that Wednesday afternoon I was in Sydney having found my way to the now all-too-familiar Westmead hospital via a taxi. The interesting thing about islet cell transplantation is that you are not under such a short timeline as for other organ donations. This is because once donated the pancreas needs to be prepared and the islets removed and then given time to determine if they are going to settle and be suitable for transplantation. This is not as time critical as a whole organ transplant and so we have time on our side with islets. I was therefore not "rushed" to the hospital like you see in the movies or escorted off the plane but made my own way via a taxi and reported to the transplant coordinator for bloods and a couple of other tests before everything began in earnest.

One of the first recollections I have is standing in the corridor with my suitcase and one of the nurses being super critical of its size! I thought I had done well given I had one suitcase for a whole month! People are so quick to judge when they do not know someone's situation. Given my family and friends are all based in South Australia, and I was going to be in New South Wales for over a month for recovery after the operation, I had packed for that entire time, knowing I would not have any visitors or much to do. I also knew I did not have anyone to bring more supplies every day and so had packed books to read and a laptop to keep me entertained.

By mid afternoon I was being prepped for a central line. In order that the islet cells had the best chance to infuse and attach to the liver, my immune system had to be weakened. The medicines that do this are very irritating and need to be delivered to the body via a large artery and not small veins like normal medicines where blood is usually extracted. And so, a central line, or catheter, was inserted in the right side of my neck. However, given the fact I had been what they describe "nil by mouth" or no fluids or food since my phone call, I had started to dehydrate. This meant all my veins and arteries were hard to find and even harder to insert a catheter in to. After the seventh try, the doctor finally managed to insert it in the eighth attempt. And despite local anaesthetic, and the doctor insisting I could not feel anything I counted every single time she tried, becoming even more impatient with each go. Having a sharp knife and then a needle in your neck once or twice is not very pleasant but let me tell you, eight times when you can feel it each time (and they kept telling me that I should not be able to) is not at all what I call fun!

I had never experienced migraines before the first transplant, although knew the effects of them due to my brother, Damien who used to have migraines as a child.

My first migraine attack began that night and lasted approximately two hours until I vomited, which allowed it to resolve. I have now had severe excruciating migraine attacks since the central line was placed in my neck and take medicine each day to manage them.

Thursday morning is a complete blur to me. I am told I went to surgery at approximately 2 pm on May 31st, 2007, where it is estimated I received approximately 450,000 islet cells. I was then "specialled" or confined to one room with its own air supply and own nurse. This happens with all transplant recipients to protect them while their bodies rebuild their depleted immune system.

When I entered the transplant program, Westmead in Sydney was the only unit in Australia performing islet cell transplants. There are two ways to transplant islet cells into the portal vein of the liver. One is to find the vein via ultrasound and then inject the cells through the skin guided by ultrasound imaging. Unfortunately, the ultrasound guided treatment was not Westmead's preferred option. I therefore required "keyhole" surgery to actually find the portal vein and inject the islets while the portal vein was exposed. Westmead liver surgeons decided this was a much safer way to ensure the trans-planted cells were deposited exactly where they were supposed to go, and I respected that decision. What I am not entirely sure of is the word "keyhole" due to the fact it must have been a big key and door given the size of the cut in my stomach!

The first proper recollection I have after the operation is Friday morning waking up after my operation in a room by myself with my own nurse, a catheter in and several IVs attached giving me fluids and pain relief.

While in reasonable pain from the cut, I have never been one to lie around in a bed, even when in hospital. In fact, I remember contracting German Measles in year 8 of high school and still not being fully aware of the consequences of contagious diseases, I hid my spots from my parents for four days because I knew I would have to stay home from school! It was only after the spots appeared on my face that my mum became aware that I had something going on and demanded to see my stomach and back!

And so, despite being attached to numerous cords, drips, and lines, I asked the nurse sitting beside my bed if I could get up and have a shower. While a little suspicious that I really would be able to manage this alone, she did not object, but did explain that I needed to be careful and to call her immediately if I felt unwell.

I credit Bikram Yoga for my physical condition and strength leading up to that first islet transplant. I had spent almost two years working on weight, and health, as much as humanly possible. And as much as my diabetes would allow. So, while I did feel lightheaded from the combination of medicines I was receiving for pain, and to reduce my immune system, I was able to shower independently and be sitting up in bed chatting away (probably not making one bit of sense mind you!) when my transplant team walked in less than 12 hours after completion of my operation. Of course, I do not remember all that were present there that Friday morning, I only remember my two main specialists in charge of my care throughout the main workup and post-transplant.

The team had come to tell me my transplant had been a success! It was estimated anywhere from 400,000-500,000 islet cells were successfully isolated and transplanted into my portal vein. Over the next week they would slowly start to produce their own insulin (which could be detected by measuring what is known as C-peptide levels). Over the next three months they would slowly and gradually produce more and more insulin, allowing me to reduce the amount of external insulin I was administering via my pump. So, my job over the next seven to ten days? To try and keep my glucose levels as close to target as possible to protect the newly transplanted cells.

Irony all over again! One of the most toxic situations for islet cells is above target glucose levels. While the primary aim of islet cell transplantation is to always reduce, and ultimately prevent hypoglycaemic unawareness, to transplant enough working cells to render an individual "insulin free" becomes a secondary goal. This is because self regulating islets, that is islets that can "turn on and turn off" insulin production so the glucose levels are never above target, will, in theory last much, much longer. The other incredibly ironic twist in islet transplantation is the anti-rejection medicines used to protect them from an individual's immune system, can eventually be toxic to them, causing long term damage. However, I take the opinion that you work with the technology you have at the time you have it.

Right, seven to ten days of perfect glucose levels. I will do my best! The problem with that once again was that I got it, but it seemed like there were many other individuals not on board with this!

Having been fasting since Wednesday and it now being Friday night and actually feeling quite well, I was hungry. I had had my insulin pump removed during surgery (standard procedure) and was now hooked up to an IV insulin infusion that was taking over the BASAL job of the pump. I enquired about having something to eat and was told that would be a fantastic idea and that I should try some toast. Great, I thought, just what I felt like. What about having some insulin (bolus dose) to cover the carbohydrates? I was then informed, quite condescendingly by some of the nursing team, that I did not need insulin anymore because I had had a pancreas transplant. They continued to explain that they understood that this was all very foreign to me, and it might take me "a couple of days to get used to my new lifestyle". Hmm ok. When entering the transplant program, I had had it explained that this was a very new procedure and that this type of confusion may occur! In fact, I had it stressed to me to make sure when I was flown and arrived in Sydney that it was understood, I was not coming for a kidney transplant. Kidney specialists have the most experience and knowledge with medicines used for islet protection and therefore I spent much time in that ward. However, I needed to be very clear that this was not what I was on the kidney ward for and that I needed to make sure others were clear about this. Right. Obviously, I needed to also be quite clear as to how much of the organ I had had transplanted and in what time frame this would begin to work! So, let's approach this a different way. Let's try speaking with my specialists about how much insulin I should give myself with two pieces of toast and where I should get that insulin from, given I had been detached from my pump and IV pumps can only mimic basal and not bolus insulin (insulin for food). Oh crap, they were all on a plane flying overseas for a transplant meeting! Great!

Unfortunately, there was absolutely no give from the nursing team at all regarding the acceptance that I might need insulin with two slices of toast. The unfortunate issue was I was in a ward where the nursing team had only ever some across full pancreas transplants. A transplanted pancreas produces insulin immediately after the operation. When a person first starts eating after surgery, they generally do not need insulin even if they required it before surgery. The issue for me was that I had not had a full pancreas transplant and I was one of the first in Australia to have an islet cell transplant so I was still reliant on my cells "waking up" after their surgery which I had been told could be three months. However, the medical team left to look after me after my surgery did not comprehend this and continued to insist that I did not need insulin with any meal. It is once again the fact I take ownership for my own health, took a strong interest in the procedure, and am blessed with intelligence and common sense that I understood I did not just have to accept what I was being told. Especially when I knew it was going to be severely detrimental to these transplanted cells if I ate toast without some form of short acting insulin. And so, a compromise if you could call it that, was reached. I agreed to eat one slice of toast as long as the nursing team promised faithfully, they would monitor my blood glucose levels every 20 minutes (I was unable to do this myself because I was still strapped to many IVs and confined to the bed) and they were to immediately ring anyone who was able to order a dose of bolus insulin as soon as my glucose level rose above 15 mmol/L (set as the level to try not to get above by the transplant team).

Within an hour of eating one slice of toast (and despite being incredibly hungry having not eaten for two days, I did not enjoy it as much as I thought due to the concern over my glucose levels), my results began to rise. Within two hours they were 17 mmol/L. This really was one of the times in my life I did not want to be right!

However, I had learnt long ago that I knew my body reasonably well and although I rarely was able to change anything, once again I had predicted above target results. And now I had all the transplant nurses in a panic! What we they going to do??? Not to be sarcastic but some insulin with food would be a start, wouldn't it? And so, after many phone calls trying to contact anyone who was able to make a decision about insulin doses, I finally got what I had been asking for and should have received with my toast, a BOLUS dose of insulin. There are pitfalls to being the first islet cell recipient in Australia! Needless to say, my insulin pump was returned soon after that Friday and I was able to deliver my own insulin for food while remaining in hospital.

I remained in the "specialled" room for only four days but having deemed me well enough to be discharged, I was then sent to Casuarina Lodge to recover from surgery.

This lodge is situated on the grounds of the Westmead hospital and is designed to help those who are living far away from the hospital. The rooms are small but are equipped with two single beds, a fridge, and a TV. There is a share bathroom and kitchen, so it really has everything that you need. More importantly, it is situated close to the transplant ward, which I found later to be especially important.

While there was an enormous amount of psychological focus prior to the procedure to determine if I was able to withstand the rigors of transplantation and all that this involved, I discovered after the event, little consideration went in to how I felt, how I was coping, and what was going on for me.

I had spent three to four years waiting for THE phone call. During that time, I tried to do everything I could to be at the peak of my fitness. While severe and regular hypoglycaemic events hindered my efforts, I regularly attended Bikram, had lost and maintained the weight the transplant team had suggested would be best and had maintained a healthy diet.

Suddenly I had dropped from my peak of fitness to being unwell. I had an exceptionally large wound across my stomach, and I felt like I had the flu. And not just a head cold like people say when they think they have the flu. Actual influenza! Every morning the sheets in my bed at the lodge were soaked in sweat, I had a fever, ached all over and had a hacking cough that hurt every time I tried to clear fluid off my chest. And yet each morning I had to get out of bed and "report" to the transplant doctors in the hospital where they would examine me, run a heap of blood tests and make sure my anti-rejection medicine dose was correct.

At one point, unable to sit on the uncomfortable chairs that reminded me of school days, I simply lay down on the filthy carpet. I was simply unable to hold my head up, let alone sit up, any longer.

Once again, my parents supported me all the way. Not only did they fly from Port Lincoln to Sydney within days of my transplant but stayed with me at Casuarina Lodge throughout my time there, looking after me. Each morning Mum stripped my bed and washed the sheets so that they were clean for the following night. Each morning one of them would accompany me to the transplant ward and sit patiently with me, sometimes for hours, while we waited for the doctor to view the day's blood results. They cooked for me and tried to interest me in food.

Unfortunately, both the anti-rejection medication and the fevers made me too ill too even think about eating or drinking. Yet they still encouraged me to try to consume nutrients.

After about a week of feeling extremely unhuman, a couple of IV bags of saline for rehydration and a chest X-Ray to ensure I did not have pneumonia, I started to feel like I was on the mend.

And then came the realisation that I had another person's cells inside my own body. Fortunately, hours of psychological counselling had at least prepared me for this moment.

I will forever be grateful for the family and loved ones who made the decision to donate organs that allowed me to receive an islet cell transplant. I cannot even begin to imagine how they felt and how hard that decision would have been. I will forever be in their debt.

What counselling did not really prepare me for is what I can only describe as a form of transference.

Having never been a fond lover a potato crisps, I suddenly, after starting to feel better, found myself craving packets of Doritos. The more I ate the more I craved. And while I did my best not to give in, the urge was almost impossible. Having lost so much weight after surgery, and not having that much of an appetite, I think Mum and Dad were just relieved to see me eating anything. Also, for some weeks after the transplant, I woke up every night at exactly 3 am. I do not know what woke me and often it was completely silent at Casuarina Lodge. Often, I had horrendous nightmares of violent car accidents around this time of the morning as well which makes me wonder about the circumstances of the death of my donor. These dreams and the waking in the early hours of the morning lasted a couple of months. The cravings for potato chips, especially Doritos has never gone away. That has remained with me until this day!

It is difficult to imagine and even more difficult if you have not had the experience to believe the concept of transference. Yet many recipients experience it. In fact, I overheard a young man who had had a kidney transplant telling other recipients he passionately believed he had received a kidney from a female donor because he had a craving for Kahlua and milk after recovery!

There are also documented changes in personality as well as preferences to music, recreation, and sex after transplantation of organs. Two of the most interesting cases I have read about is that of heart transplant recipient Claire Sylvia and Demi-Lee who was an Australian who received a liver transplant.

Claire began getting cravings for beer and KFC's chicken nuggets, things she says she did not eat before her surgery and in line with what I say about Doritos. She also started having vivid dreams about a man named "Tim L". Upon further research she was able to identify her donor and the foods she craved were named, by Tim's family, as some of his favourite.

Demi-Lee received a liver transplant and after just nine months had changed blood type to that of her donor.

There are many theories where scientists will try to explain how transference occurs. I am comfortable with "cellular memory". Each organ (or in my case a mass of cells) do not exist independently of the rest of an individual. When that organ is generously donated to another individual, the experiences, personality, and everything that makes that person unique is transferred with that part of the body. I accept the gift in its entirety. I am unable to answer why transference does not occur with all transplants except to say that it may be as much about the donor as the recipient's ability to receive.

Three weeks of rest and recuperation, eating Doritos and toasted ham and cheese sandwiches (my food of choice when I do not feel overly well) and I felt like I was ready for home. How much tougher it is to be in another state away from your own bed, friends, and family! While I was under no illusion that I was going to be going out socialising, I found myself incredibly lonely. While I continued to remind myself it was not forever, it was a tough three weeks. Finally, it was looking like I could pack up and fly home.

Before doing this however Mum, Dad and I decided we would visit Taronga Zoo for the day out. Having visited the transplant clinic in the morning and been given all clear, we set off via the trains.

Halfway to the centre of Sydney however I started to lose my vision. Having had retinopathy for a number of years and fluctuating glucose levels that affected my vision quite significantly, I was not too concerned when this first presented itself. Checking my glucose result to ensure I was not dropping low, I noted my level was within target range. And then the second of my migraines hit.

Noticing something wrong Mum asked what was going on. Sitting on a packed and cramped train at least half an hour from the hospital with a pounding headache, I was almost unable to communicate. Yet somehow, I managed to let my parents know that I needed to get off the train, on to one heading back to Westmead and get to Casuarina Lodge before throwing up everywhere.

How I managed this I do not really know. I do not remember the train ride back, but I do remember the walk from the train station as every step made my head pound even more. Crawling into my bed at Casuarina I managed to mumble to my Mum to ask her to ring the hospital before closing my eyes and hoping I would die so the pain would just stop. Within what seemed like a few moments one of the nurses from the transplant clinic had appeared in my room with a wheelchair to take me into the hospital: the advantages of the proximity of the lodge. I guess flying home was out of the question, right? Not that I really cared at that present moment.

One of the worries of being immunocompromised is that I was more susceptible to life-threatening organisms such as meningitis. This is what was suspected given the extreme symptoms of headache and vomiting. I was given strong pain relief and admitted for close observation in hospital.

My headache and vomiting went on for four days. At one point I remember begging the doctors to make my headache stop. Nothing seemed to be working. While everything sinister like meningitis had been ruled out, a reason for my severe headaches could not be found.

On the fifth day I refused pain relief. It seemed each time I took more pain relief, I vomited. Each time I vomited, it set off my migraine. Nausea and vomiting can be side effects of some of the stronger pain medicines. Understanding this, I decided I was prepared, at this point, to have a day without them. Using whatever tactics I had, deep breathing and visualisation, I spent most of the day and night drifting in and out of sleep to wake up the next day headache free.

Not wanting to experience that again, I had agreed on migraine prevention medication and, armed with this, felt confident to return to South Australia.

CHAPTER 9

Home Sweet Home

How nice to be home in my own bed. How nice to wake up in my own house and to go outside and pat my dogs when I woke up. Sitting down to breakfast on the first day home, I suddenly realised how tired I was. At least I could spend time in my own house resting after the trip back. There is not enough emphasis given, in my opinion, to the benefits of being surrounded by positive energy and love. I immediately felt better, being surrounded by my own comforts, with my animals and in my home state. I no longer felt as isolated and so far away from all those I cared about and loved. While Casuarina Lodge was comfortable and provided what I needed to recover from my surgery, there was nothing quite like being where I wanted to be.

Unfortunately, this was not to be the case for long. My third migraine attack hit within hours of waking up on my first morning home from Sydney. And this was worse than the other two attacks and required an ambulance trip to the Queen Elizabeth Hospital in Adelaide.

When first being chosen as a candidate for an islet transplant, only Westmead hospital in Sydney was involved. However, in 2006 the then Minister for Health and Ageing, Tony Abbott, announced $30 million towards the Islet Transplantation Program, in collaboration with JDRF. This meant centres at not only Westmead but also St Vincent's hospital in Melbourne and the Queen Elizabeth Hospital (which was later moved to the Royal Adelaide Hospital and called the South Australian and Northern Territory Islet Program SANTIP) in South Australia.

While I was officially considered a transplant patient of the Westmead team, it did mean that I had another amazing team close to home in my own state that I was able to see and have regular check ups with.

And so, despite having a referral from Westmead and an action plan to catch up with the Adelaide team at some stage upon my return into the state, this happened a little too quickly for my liking!

And so off to the Queen Elizabeth Hospital via ambulance where I spent three more days with severe vomiting and my head feeling like it was being spit open with an axe. And again, despite numerous tests and scans, no cause was found. I was released once the pain lessened and the headache resolved to again begin my rest and healing period at home. Oh well, at least I got to meet the Adelaide transplant team, albeit much quicker than first anticipated!

Over the next three months I started, ironically, to have more hypoglycaemic episodes straight after administering a bolus dose of insulin with a meal. This was the beginning of the transplanted cells starting to produce reasonable amounts of endogenous (meaning coming from internally; the transplanted cells) insulin in response to the food that I had eaten. And so, I began to give less and less insulin from my pump with each meal. The most exciting thing of all was that once I began reducing my insulin from my pump, my hypos began reducing significantly until they stopped all together! For the first time in years, I felt safe. Safe from hypos at night even. The first objective of islet cell transplantation had proven successful. Resolution from hypoglycaemia. All hypoglycaemia!

The trade off? Anti-rejection medications and their gamut of side effects. As a health professional, I understand that all medicines we take, regardless of what they are and what we take them for, have some adverse effects. We, as individuals, need to make decisions as to whether the benefits outweigh the negative impacts. Sometimes the decision to change or stop medication, in consultation with a health care team, may be straightforward.

Obviously with anti-rejection medicine it is not that simple. Stopping would mean my transplanted islet cells would reject due to my immune system recognising them as foreign.

I went into the transplant in what I believed was my peak physical condition, albeit with type 1 diabetes, retinopathy, and hypoglycaemic unawareness. However, I now had swapped these conditions with the side effects of two medicines, mycophenolate and tacrolimus.

Early efforts of transplantation of islets, and that of most whole organ transplants, required the use of glucocorticoid immunosuppressants as anti-rejection medication. James Shapiro and Jonathan Lakey made a discovery while working at the University of Alberta, Edmonton, which they developed into the "Edmonton protocol". Shapiro and Lakey revolutionised islet cell transplantation by successfully transplanting without glucocorticoids, which, long term, are toxic to the very cells they are trying to protect.

Without glucocorticoid immunosuppressants the remaining anti-rejection medicines available were much less "diabetes toxic long term". As stated previously, glucocorticoid immunosuppressants can cause insulin resistance long term which can cause steroid induced diabetes. This is the irony of using steroids in both pancreas and islet cell transplants. The Edmond protocol revolutionised this.

Mycophenolate prevents B and T cells from forming in the bone marrow (they are responsible for "finding and eating" bacteria and viruses). They are also responsible for recognising cancer in your body. Tacrolimus works more specifically on the T cells in the immune system, preventing them from becoming specialised to "home in" on molecules recognised by our immune system. However, mycophenolate, tacrolimus and sirolimus are still not without side effects.

While I was able to get away with much smaller doses than an individual with a whole organ transplant, I was not able to escape without considerable side effects.

These included severe diarrhoea, fast heartbeat, extreme fatigue and weight loss (mycophenolate) and tremor, abnormal dreams, flu-like symptoms, tremor (of hands which was noticeable), flushing of face and neck (this happened between 2-4 pm every day), and joint pain (courtesy of tacrolimus).

Working in a rather public profession in a regional setting there was considerable interest from the general community about my islet transplant. One of the most interesting things I learnt on my transplant journey was the revelation of how other people perceived my diabetes. Interestingly there were many comments along the lines of "I did not realise just how sick you were". It was only after the fourth or fifth person made such a comment that I took notice of exactly what they were saying.

I had, and still do not, consider myself "sick". I have a chronic health condition and, although extremely challenging at times, I believe I lead a full and healthy life with what I've got. "Sick" or "unwell" are never words I would use to describe myself. Nor has it ever occurred to me to do so; even faced with all the challenges of the transplant and the side effects of the medicine I took to prevent the rejection of the transplanted islet cells. And yet suddenly I was faced with the perception that that was how others viewed me. This did not bother me in the slightest, nor impact me in any way. I just found it interesting and something I had never considered before!

Having recovered from one transplant, I decided it would be sensible to begin trying to improve my physical fitness again, especially if I was to have a second transplant. What better way than to get back into Bikram Yoga and to start doing the things I loved? Unfortunately, my mind was willing, but my body not so able! I am not even sure I lasted the whole 90 minutes of the whole class when I went back for my first yoga after the transplant. While I had enjoyed the heat and the extra flexibility it allowed before the surgery, afterwards I was simply unable to tolerate it. Unfortunately for now Bikram would have to wait.

Instead, I decided to get bike fit for the next JDRF Ride to Cure Diabetes that was coming up in January. Checking my glucose level before setting off (yep, within target) I rode along a bike track near my house for about 5 kms before stopping for a quick rest and a drink of water. Another check of my glucose level (still in target range) and feeling very, very tired but pleased with my efforts, I set off for home.

While the bike track is relatively flat, there were some slight hills on the way home. What surprised me significantly was the fact that I was unable to pedal up these slight hills at all! In fact, I was barely able to walk up them! Suddenly I was out of breath, fatigued and the more I tried to get back on my bike the worse my symptoms got. At one point I did wonder if I was having a panic attack, so extreme was my inability to breathe. Having spent approximately one hour cycling down the bike track, it now took me twice as long to get home! And when I did finally arrive, I was exhausted.

As luck would have it, the following day, I saw both my endocrinologist and the transplant team for my regular checks to ensure islets were functioning well. Having mentioned the bike ride, extra blood tests were taken to determine why I felt so extraordinarily exhausted while riding. The result? Severe anaemia. Not enough iron in my blood to carry the oxygen around. Well, that explained all my symptoms then. And unfortunately, another side effect of the anti-rejection medicine. And so I would now need regular iron infusions to counteract this side effect. Nonetheless this was a small price to pay if it meant that I was going to be completely hypoglycaemia free.

And so, without the constant worry of hypos on considerably less insulin per day, and with the trade-off of multiple side effects from the anti-rejection medicines, I entered a new era in my health journey.

CHAPTER 10

There Is No Such Thing As A Diabetic!

Whilst transitioning through all the islet cell transplants and getting to know a new way of life, I decided to change direction in my career.

Having always worked in the health industry as a community pharmacist and been heavily involved with people with diabetes through supply of their medication, and NDSS (National Diabetes Services Scheme), many of the customers at the local pharmacy where I worked often asked me questions about their diabetes. Having an intimate knowledge of how medicines work from a pharmaceutical perspective was one thing. However, I decided to expand my knowledge and, via correspondence, completed my Graduate Certificate in Diabetes Education through Curtin University in Western Australia. I was now a diabetes educator as well as a pharmacist.

Unfortunately, the more I began working in the industry, the more I began to understand how complex and complicated the industry was.

To become a diabetes educator, a health care professional must complete a one-year post-graduate course; in my case, this was the course I completed through Curtin University. A higher level of endorsement, known as being a Credentialled Diabetes Educator

(CDE) can then be gained through the Australian Diabetes Educators Association (ADEA). This acknowledges the educator's ongoing study and accumulated hours of experience from working as a diabetes educator. Being credentialled allows an educator to charge Medicare, Veteran's Affairs and private health insurance funds to assist a person with diabetes. The problem for me when I first qualified as an educator was that the hours supporting people with diabetes while working as a pharmacist were not recognised by the ADEA towards becoming credentialled.

This was something I simply could not understand. Or accept.

I was a health professional, and I had studied and passed the post graduate diabetes education course. Why was it that pharmacists could not be recognised as credentialled diabetes educators? Pharmacists have a bachelor's degree in medicines and while medication is certainly not the only way we address islet cell, and therefore, insulin, depletion, it is one of the mainstays with which we continue to treat all forms of diabetes. Surely if there was scope for other health care professionals to become educators, there was scope for pharmacists to be credentialled as well, providing the correct study was undertaken?

And so, it began. And continued. In 2008, to gain more experience as an educator, and to gain experience in a multidisciplinary team, I joined Diabetes South Australia (current trading name is Diabetes SA but formerly known as The Diabetic Association of South Australia) and worked part time there and part time in pharmacy and, despite many hurdles, gained my credentialled status later that same year. I was the first pharmacist to be a credentialled diabetes educator in Australia.

While this is something I am proud of, it is not the reason I pushed ahead to become credentialled. The reason I did this is multi-layered. One of the major reasons to be honest was because I was told I was not able to! I really do not like to be told no. It makes me more determined to do something, especially if I believe it is right and, in this case, I believe it was! I had heard along the "grapevine" that it was the opinion of some of my fellow colleagues who were credentialled educators that individuals with diabetes "shouldn't be educators". Again, this is not something that I necessarily agree with. This is a generalised, broad statement that has no basis. I have a sound background and knowledge in health. I also have experience living with diabetes. That experience allows me to empathise much better with my clients. Not sympathise. But show empathy. Having lived with type 1 diabetes for many years before choosing this as a career allows great insight that gives me an advantage that others may not have. I believe that makes me better at what I do every single day. The other reason I believe some pharmacists make good diabetes educators is that we play an important role in the health care team and, on average, see the public with health care conditions approximately fourteen times more in any one year than other health care professionals. Pharmacists are also the most accessible health care professional. This has its positives and negatives. Whilst it often holds up the prescription wait time considerably if we get caught in a long explanation with a person with complex needs, the proximity does allow for the ability for anyone to ask questions easily and have access to answers when they require help.

Once I joined the extended health care team at Diabetes SA, I expanded my book knowledge and my own experience tremendously working alongside an incredibly supportive care team. I also gained confidence as a guest speaker and learnt ways to impart the knowledge I had in an easy way so that others would understand what their health condition meant to them.

One of the other most important insights I learnt while working at Diabetes SA was regarding wording and mental health. Diabetes Australia had released a position statement suggesting that health professionals should be mindful of the words used to not only describe a person with diabetes but also all the technology we use to help treat this condition. People lose their identity and BECOME the HEALTH CONDITION, which impacts significantly on mental health, family units, relationships, work and almost every aspect of that person's life. This, in turn, can have a negative effect on that person's diabetes, making an individual feel de-motivated and less empowered. And yet language is so underrated. After I became aware of the position statement, I began to become much more mindful of the impact language has both in a positive and negative manner. While ingrained in our everyday speech, what is often overlooked is how language can have far reaching consequences.

From the moment I was diagnosed with diabetes, I understood I had to live with a chronic health condition. Yet never was I treated as "sick" by my parents. I am also not a "diabetic" because I am not a disease state. I am an individual who happens to have diabetes. I do not "test", I monitor (and there is no pass or fail with the number that appears on the blood glucose machine). It is, after all just a number, and while I do my best to hit the target range, it is not always possible to achieve levels in the target range. There is also no diabetes "control" (as if I have any of that!). There is however management.

Words, attitude, and judgement are so important. It was when this position statement was released, and I had the privilege of reading it that I had my "AH-HA" moment. It was at that moment I truly began to understand the nature of my relationship with my diabetes and what it had meant to me for all these years. Due to the words that had been used to describe my diabetes as a young child I had grown up thinking that my diabetes was my fault, that the fluctuating glucose levels and elevated HbA1cs were under "my control" and any results that were not in target were always because I had done something wrong. However, I did not really understand all these feelings until I read the position statement. Although as an adult I understood that I did not have complete ability to manage every single component of my diabetes, I did everything humanly possible to follow what my health care team had asked of me, especially in the early stages of my diagnosis. And yet still I was blamed for glucose levels not in target, weight gain, weight loss, skipping insulin doses, eating the "wrong" foods, not eating the "right" foods, not exercising enough, not doing enough glucose "tests', eating in the middle of the night (later it was discovered that this was due to dawn phenomenon) -everything was blamed on me!

While the language position statement did not solve my fluctuating glucose levels, what it did for me was allow me the ability to articulate that my diabetes is one part of me and not the whole of me! It is not my whole identity, and it is not my everything! It is not me! And I am not it! I have a chronic health condition that is hard work and that takes a whole health care team (who I have hand selected) to manage.

It has taken me many years and a slight change in my career path to understand this and realise the importance of mindfulness. Once I came to this realisation, I was better able to accept that I could not control every outcome and every blood glucose level. I have come to realise, over time that while I am very proactive with almost every area in my life, type 1 diabetes is not an area that I can be as proactive as I would like to be. Rather diabetes can cause frustration for me due to needing to be reactive to a degree.

I now challenge individuals each day to be not only be aware of language but mindful of the concept that we should never treat an individual as a health condition. They are first and foremost an individual. They simply happen to have a medical condition This is important not only for diabetes but for all chronic health conditions. No one should ever be defined by a disease!

A copy of the position statement can be found here: https://www.diabetesaustralia.com.au/wp-content/uploads/Language-Matters-2021-Diabetes-Australia-Position-Statement-1.pdf

CHAPTER 11

Chocolate and Red Wine

It is estimated an individual needs approximately one million islet cells for insulin independence. At transplant one I received approximately 500,000 cells. So, I required a second islet transplant to be free of my pump, but more importantly to allow the cells producing insulin to self regulate. Self regulation means the cells will, in theory, survive much longer as they have their own ability to protect themselves against above target glucose levels.

Having been accepted into the islet cell transplant program I had always known there would be two transplants. What I had not been prepared for was how hard recovery from the medication and side effects from the first transplant would be. What is also extremely difficult is the mental strength required. Having no idea what I was in for the first time around made things so much easier. The saying "ignorance is bliss" certainly applied when describing me when I agreed for the first transplant.

What I also found challenging was the overwhelming feelings of guilt that I experienced after the first transplant. I will always, always be eternally grateful for the enormous generosity of the families who choose to donate organs of their loved ones. This is the most amazing gift. Thank you to anyone who chooses to be an organ donor and to the amazing families who honour the gift of a loved one at one of the hardest and saddest times of their families' lives.

However, after the first transplant, I found it difficult when strangers kept telling me that I "must feel grateful that I had received donated islet cells". Please do not misinterpret this. I was eternally grateful for this generous gift. However, I was not grateful to be in the situation where I needed them in the first place! I hated having to be in such desperate need that I had run out of every other option and was now at the point that I required not only one transplant but two! I was exhausted from the procedure, incredibly sick from the medicines to prevent the islet cells rejecting, and anxious that I had to do it all over again! And quite frankly I was a little tired of strangers telling me I should feel grateful! Would they feel that way?

What compounded my feelings was the inability to have a platform to express my real feelings. That and the fact that every time I felt this way, I then felt incredibly guilty, because common sense "told" me that, of course I should feel grateful! An enormous amount of counselling before the first transplant did not prepare me for the fact, I would have complete strangers telling me how to feel at almost every second of every day!

Despite this, and despite all the anxiety and anticipation, a second transplant was planned. So back to being on call, although this time I was promised quite a short wait list because the aim was to get as many functioning islet cells transplanted so they were "self regulating" and therefore "self protecting". On the 7th of April 2008 I received another phone call regarding flying back to Sydney for a second transplant. To be honest I have little, if any recollection of this call, and certainly not the vivid recall I had of the first one! This may have had much to do with the fact that during the time between the first and second transplant I had been on many failed trips back and forth to Sydney in the hope of receiving more islet cells.

This meant packing a bag, flying over, and waiting around in the hospital sitting room, often for up to eight to ten hours, for a determination to be made as to whether the donated cells were viable for transplantation. By viable, it means that they had survived the isolation process so that they could potentially survive the transplantation process. While eight to ten hours does not seem all that long from a time perspective, it is a considerably long time when you are not able to eat or drink anything in case of surgery. Then the seconds tick away very very slowly.

So, on multiple occasions, I flew to Sydney, waited for many hours in the fasting state, only to be sent home to await a further phone call. When the call came on the 7th of April, I was already in the swing of flying interstate and quite familiar with the trip to Westmead. This phone call therefore did not feel all that different to many of the other phone calls that I had received in the eleven months I had been back on the waiting list.

Once again, the work up began in preparation for the transplantation of the generously donated islet cells. Again, I was required to have a whole gamut of medication to deplete my immune system to prevent my body rejecting newly introduced cells. However, this time I refused to have a central line inserted. While I understood the importance of reducing any chance the implanted cells could be rejected, I was simply unable to have another central line inserted after the trauma of the last time (or eight times but who's counting!!). Instead, I chose to have the anti-rejection cocktail administered via a PICC (peripherally inserted central catheter) line in my arm. While again extremely uncomfortable, it was still a much more tolerable experience than the central line in my neck that occurred with the first transplant.

Following all the preparation, blood work and tests, on the 8th of April 2008, I received my second transplant of insulin producing cells. I also began experiencing transference all over again.

Having been so unwell with the immunosuppressant medication with the first transplant, and unable, despite all good intentions, to do any form of daily physical activity, it left me very much unprepared for the second transplant from a physical and mental health perspective. And so, having bounced out of bed 24 hours after "keyhole surgery" I did not the second time around.

This time around, I had severe side effects from the medicine given to me to relieve the pain from the surgery. Once again, I had days of extreme nausea and vomiting, this time from the surgery rather than from migraines. However, despite severe vomiting in hospital, I had unreasonable cravings for red wine and chocolate at the same time! I have absolutely no doubt that I would not have been able to eat these at the time, especially while throwing up but it did not stop me having a strong desire for them.

Great, more food cravings. Doritos, chocolate, and red wine! Boy, was I going to give the transplanted islet cells a workout if I ever did become insulin independent! This was however all I noticed from the second donor. There were no dreams, and the red wine and chocolate liking was not as strong as the Doritos. So again, while I have no ability to know any details about my second donor, I believe this person was female. While a generalisation, it seems to me that more females than males are inclined to enjoy such foods as wine and chocolate.

Once again over the time frame of three to four weeks, with plenty of rest and support from my amazing family, friends, and the transplant team, I began the process of regaining my strength after surgery and began the wait for the new transplanted mass of islet cells to begin to function at full potential.

When feeling well enough and once again being given the all clear to fly back to South Australia and return to work, it soon became obvious the transplanted cells had begun to produce insulin.

Over the course of a month or so after the second transplant, I began to have hypoglycaemic episodes once again. In fact, one day, walking to work I remember feeling very unsteady on my feet. Stopping to check my glucose level, it was 1.3 mmol/L. Ok that is very much under 4 mmol/L! And so, I knew it had begun. Slowly but surely the second phase of the reduction of my total daily insulin dose began. I began to reduce my basal rate over the course of the following month until I had lowered the basal rate to approximately 25 units a day. While this is still quite a bit of insulin for some individuals, for me, this was almost a quarter of the total daily dose of what I had been on before the transplants. More importantly, my glucose levels did not shift whenever I checked them. They hovered consistently around 5 mmol/L, and again all hypoglycaemic episodes had ceased!

CHAPTER 12

Round Three

Over time, despite my drop in weight before beginning the islet cell transplants it gradually became obvious that I was not able to become insulin independent on two transplants. And so began the very difficult decision as to whether a third one should be considered. Insulin independence is not the be all and end all. However self regulation of the islet helps the transplanted cells survive long term. This is the only reason I agreed to a third transplant, especially knowing about the procedure and how difficult recovery was.

On Saturday 6th September 2008, I received my third lot of transplanted islet cells. As I had been leaving work on Friday 5th I realised I had missed four calls from Sydney Westmead. I had turned my phone to silent while presenting at work and forgotten to turn the ring tone back on. Oops! Nonetheless I managed to get hold of the transplant co-ordinator immediately upon this realisation and was still able to organise and catch an early flight on the Saturday morning. I then had surgery that same day.

This time no central or PICC line. Yay. This was because my immune system was already low enough, and the decision was made that my immune system was potentially not an enormous threat for newly transplanted cells. However, I did still need "keyhole" surgery to ensure the donated cells were placed correctly in the portal vein of the liver. And there was still lots of pain from this procedure and numerous side effects from the pain modifiers given after the surgery.

Given the amount of severe nausea and vomiting from traditional medicines such as morphine and codeine that I had experienced in the past two transplants, the specialists had chosen not to use these and instead to use one called ketamine (known as "Special K" when obtained illegally). While it certainly helped my pain without the nausea, I had unbearable head spins, hallucinations, and vivid dreams. I also tried to climb out of a window that faced out onto a side street two stories above street level. I remember waking up with one foot outside the window in the middle of the night (I think it was the cold air that woke me up) thinking "If I continue climbing out, how will I get back in?" Luckily the human mind works in bizarre ways sometimes because that thought probably saved me from some very nasty injuries! After that near miss, I asked to have the ketamine removed from my IV and just dealt with the pain for approximately three to four days. Much better than the side effects that I seemed so prone to!

Interestingly I had no cravings third time around. No changes in my taste buds. No dreams and nothing different at all. And as odd as this sounds, the third transplant felt different. I cannot really describe in what way or articulate why I believed the third transplant was different from the first or second, but I can only describe how I felt in the recovery period the week after the transplant. Exactly one week after the third surgery, and feeling reasonably well, I negotiated with the transplant team and was able to fly back to South Australia. Having not had a central or PICC line, and without the large quantity of anti-rejection medication, I did not need to be monitored as closely the third time round. This meant I was able to be released home much earlier.

And so we were back to the waiting game. Waiting for the newly transplanted cells to begin producing insulin. A month of waiting and nothing happened. There was no plausible reason for the third transplant not to be successful but unfortunately this was not meant to be. The third lot of transplanted islet cells did not appear to "wake up" and begin producing insulin. As previously stated, one of the current limitations of islet transplantation is how well the transplanted cells embed and survive (known as long term graft function). There was, at the time of my transplant, a reasonably new medicine released to the market for use in individuals who have type 2 diabetes known as a glucagon like peptide-1 (GLP-1) receptor agonist. Called exenatide (Byetta®). I was told it could improve the function of the islets I had had transplanted, prevent potential future loss of islet mass, and possibly even stimulate islet regeneration. Armed with this information, I agreed to try this injection twice a day, as well as run the small amount of basal insulin (now about 19 units a day) through my insulin pump and, of course, still take all the anti-rejection medicines.

Of course, once again, all medicines have side effects. Of course, I got most of them! Nausea, vomiting, weight loss, loss of appetite and diarrhoea. The irony of struggling to lose weight before the transplant was that I was now struggling to keep it on! By now had lost so much weight that my insulin sensitivity had completely changed since the start of the transplants. Given this, and with the exenatide on board, it was decided to trial a two-week period without my pump supplying basal insulin to determine if this would stimulate any dormant islet cells to produce insulin. (It was proposed that, due to the outside insulin from my pump keeping my blood glucose levels well within the healthy range, the transplanted islet cells may not be working to full capacity).

And so again some experimentation began. After years on insulin, 8 of which were on an insulin pump I stopped insulin therapy. A very bizarre feeling! And one I did not get used to for long unfortunately.

Coming off my insulin pump did trigger some above target glucose levels, although not extremely elevated due to having two lots of transplanted islets to help with these. However, the implanted mass of cells was not enough to keep my glucose levels within the healthy range without the background insulin from my pump.

What this ultimately meant was no insulin independence for me. While this was never my main objective when I considered transplantation, the concern for me was if the cells were not self regulating (managing their own rises and falls in glucose levels by turning insulin production on and off) how long would they potentially last? However, despite all my concerns about the long term and the trials that were required post third transplant, I still had no hypoglycaemic episodes and my blood glucose levels remained stable.

Life for someone with stable type 1 diabetes certainly is quite different from that of someone with unstable (or in the old terminology " brittle") diabetes. Because taking medicines to prevent rejection of the transplanted cells and the need to ensure everything was running smoothly, I admit there were far more blood tests and significantly more health appointments. But all in all, things from a health perspective had finally reached equilibrium.

CHAPTER 13

Health Equilibrium

Health equilibrium was quite simple for me. Nothing extravagant but things that others consider normal. Health is something that is very much taken for granted until an individual no longer has it. Our health system also has a focus on treating sickness rather than placing an emphasis on supporting and encouraging health. Things are changing but it is very slow. Initiatives in gym (or yoga) memberships, healthy eating incentives and stress management need priority.

For me it was little victories like walking my two beautiful dogs without planning this two hours in advance (so a temporary rate could be activated on my insulin pump), and not have to pack food and my mobile phone and letting someone know where I would be going. Now I could just go for a walk on a whim. Without planning!

That and being able to go on holidays overseas! Having stable blood glucose levels meant being able to travel feeling secure and safe. In fact one of the most memorable trips I have ever attempted was to Egypt in 2009 and, with stable glucose levels, one of the most enjoyable from a health perspective.

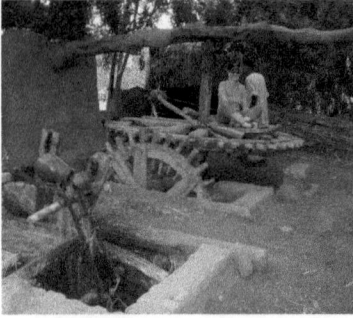

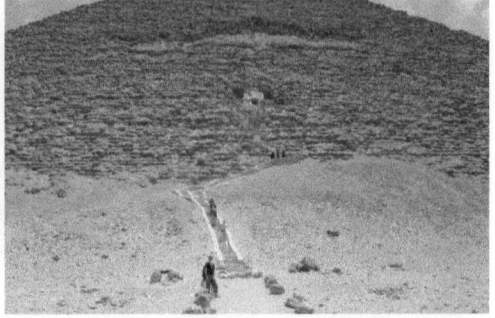

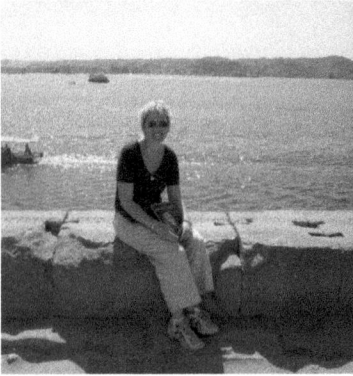

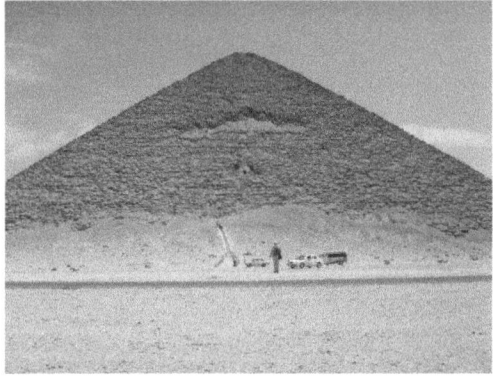

Photos of Egypt trip 2009

Having had stable glucose levels for approximately three years, I did however start to notice some fluctuations and some hypoglycaemic episodes creeping back in. While not overly concerning because they were not as low as I had had pre-transplant, there was some discussion as to whether the transplanted cells had begun to fail due to the toxicity of the anti-rejection medicines.

In 2011 I was working full time as a credentialled diabetes educator in private practice based in a pharmacy. Having learnt as much as I possibly was able in a multidisciplinary team at Diabetes South Australia I decided to resign from my position and open a private clinic, educating and empowering individuals with diabetes closer to my home in the Adelaide Hills.

The occasional hypoglycaemic episodes, however, began to occur on a more regular basis, and began to, on occasion, last longer with levels at a much lower range. And then the unthinkable happened.

There is not normally one reason for a major hypoglycaemic episode. There are usually multiple causes. Looking back on what caused my major hypo in the early hours of Monday 23rd May 2011, there were many contributing factors. The day before I had worked a 12-hour shift as a pharmacist and despite being incredibly busy, my blood glucose levels had remained above target all day. Subsequently, I had continued to give correction doses as suggested by my insulin pump. Having been concerned about what the function of the islet cells was then currently like, I made a mental note to have a discussion with the transplant team the following day during my usual monthly appointment.

Twelve-hour shifts without a break are never easy. However, I try to never let my diabetes get in the way of anything that anyone else would do. I try to be sensible and monitor often as well as eat as healthily as I can, steps I take in everyday life.

I had also recently started on a new medication and the main side effect was drowsiness. While I started on an exceptionally low dose, I had also recently lost a significant amount of weight so while the dose was very low it was still a very significant dose given my current weight. What this also meant was the side effects were potentially going to be much more pronounced for me than they would have possibly been for another individual starting them.

So above target blood glucose levels all day on Sunday 22nd requiring extra insulin, a long working day making me tired, a new medicine with a side effect of drowsiness, more stress than normal and a decent amount of weight loss causing a likely change in my insulin sensitivity were my contributing factors to the second major hypoglycaemic episode of my life.

Leaving work Sunday night at 9pm I remember very clearly arriving home and doing nothing out of the ordinary. I do remember monitoring my glucose level (9.2 mmol/L) before having a chocolate chip cookie (carbohydrate total of about 15 grams) without insulin before snuggling into bed for a well-earned rest. A quick check that I had set an early alarm (I had a 7am appointment with my transplant doctor) and finally I went to sleep!

It is at this point I would like to acknowledge all the wonderful individuals I work with and those who were involved with saving my life. It is estimated at approximately 2am Monday 23rd May 2011 my blood glucose level dipped dangerously low.

I did not go to my appointment with my transplant doctor, nor did I turn up to work on that Monday. Instead, I remained in a hypoglycaemic coma until approximately 11am when the husband of one of the team members who I work with arrived at my house (with her) and (with permission from one of my bosses) proceeded to break into my house. To say my front door was never quite the same again is possibly a considerable understatement. I will however never be able to express my gratitude that they persisted in making the decisions they did. Without their diligence, care, consideration, and refusal to just think that I simply had not turned up to work on that Monday, this book (along with many other things of course) may never have been written. Thank you.

It is also true; individuals can hear even when they are not able to respond. While I did not see lights or any tunnels while unconscious, my first recollection was my then dog Banjo barking at the paramedics. I also remember being very cold and thinking if I could just cuddle him that would stop him barking and he would keep me warm!

My next real memory was in the ambulance being transported to hospital. One of the paramedics was talking to me telling me his name was Phil. I was however incredibly frustrated because Phil (and Barb his partner who was driving the rig) were not answering any of my questions. What I did not realise at the time was that all my questions that I was asking were in my head! The only sense that had returned was my hearing! No sight, no feeling, no speech, not sure about taste! Probably a good thing it had not occurred to me that my brain was not working properly because I may have panicked!! Luckily, I was far too busy being angry at Barb and Phil for not answering my questions!!

Eventually I was able to talk. When I was able to do this, I must have asked where I was over and over. Although I have no recollection of where I was, or what had happened, I have a vague sensation of feeling that when Phil was explaining that I was in an ambulance about five minutes away from hospital having had a very severe hypoglycaemic episode, that this was not the first, second, third and would not be the last time he would say these words today. Yet he said them with patience without once making me feel like an idiot. For that I am eternally thankful.

At this point I would like to say to all emergency personal THANK YOU for all your help, patience, and service you provide to the public but especially me when I have hypoglycaemic episodes. Type 1 diabetes, and hypoglycaemia, is often very much misunderstood. However, my recollection of the care and consideration that was showed to me on the day that I had my severe hypoglycaemic episode will not be forgotten. Despite not having the ability to remember much, or, at times, speak, or even move, I do remember feeling safe and secure and not at all frightened.

Upon arriving at hospital in emergency, I was treated with more IV (intravenous) glucose and being given a range of sugary (refined) foods and complex carbohydrates in both the emergency room and in the ward. Having now gained full consciousness, although still with not much recollection, it was deemed safe for me to eat. A couple of days of being monitored by the endocrinologists in the hospital and it was deemed safe enough for me to return home.

As so there it was. Severe hypo number two. What was more significant about this one however was that the transplanted islet cells had probably failed. Although I tried (and I did my best) to convince the team both in South Australia and Westmead not to stop the anti-rejection medicine and therefore preserve any functioning islets, (realistically there were no C-peptide levels and therefore no insulin detectable in my blood) there was no convincing them after the hypoglycaemic episode that I had just had. It was reasoned that the coma could have been caused by any remaining islet cells rejecting, which released the insulin that they contained. And so, in 2011, it was deemed my transplants had stopped working, and I had stopped producing my own insulin. To keep me on the immuno-suppression medicine would just increase my long-term complication risks, including health conditions like cancer.

And so, without too much fuss (from my health care team, I must admit there was some fuss made by me!!) the immunosuppression medicine was ceased.

Did I feel any different? Not really from a diabetes perspective. Over the previous six months I had slowly but surely increased my insulin doses anyway so while I may have added a small amount of insulin once the medicines stopped, I was surprised at how little extra insulin I needed.

On a positive note, I felt much much better off all the anti-rejection medicine. I had much more energy, although I still had the occasional migraine. AND I began my beloved Bikram yoga again.

In the early stages after the failure of the transplants I was often asked if I regret having entered the islet program. Not at all. The problem I had the minute the cells began to fail was that the hypoglycaemic episodes were back. And my glucose levels were drop-ping lower and lower before I realised what was happening and I was able to treat them if at all. I was aware, going into the transplant program that it may only buy a certain amount of time so to speak. That time frame for me was four years. This seemed reasonable to me. While I had some significant side effects from the anti-rejection medicines, some complications from the surgeries and now, only after four years, faced with rejection I have absolutely no regrets. Especially given the severity of the hypoglycaemic episode I had just had. Four years is a long time to enjoy stable, predictable blood glucose levels. Four years does not seem like a long time to someone who has not lived with the unpredictability of glucose levels that I have lived with. Four years of stability for me was worth all that I sacrificed and endured. Now that was over.

Where to from here?

CHAPTER 14

Jelly Babies

To have the generosity of supportive friends who care only for your well being is a precious jewel. That is what I have in many of my very dear friends. Two very dear friends, having saved my life that Monday morning, took it upon themselves to set up a safety net in case of any further hypoglycaemic episodes. Every morning before 8am I sent them a text message so that they knew I was awake. If I did not they told me they were coming knocking on my door. This amazing hand of friendship I can never repay. It gave me some peace of mind knowing there was some back up if I did not wake up again. Knowing that individuals were willing to offer help in a way that would invade their individual space each morning, weekends and holidays included, is something I will never be able to properly express my gratitude for.

My medical team of course were also extremely concerned about the recent severe low blood glucose level and rejected islet cells. The question now was what to do given that it appeared I was back to being very unstable. While future technology looked promising, I once again needed to keep myself as well as I could until this technology "caught up" and was able to offer me a solution to both my unstable, extremely unpredictable blood glucose levels and my extreme hypoglycaemic episodes. Well, that should be reasonably easy right? Ha!

Never one to dwell too much on tasks that I do not have much control over, I turned my attention on things where I was able to have some influence.

Interestingly having entered the transplant program on what had been described as reasonably large amounts of total daily doses of insulin for my body weight, I was now on much smaller doses even though the transplanted islet cells had rejected. There was no clinical reason for this. No working islet cells in theory meant that I should be back to the same amount of insulin pre-transplant. Yet this was not the case. This went some way to reducing the swings of extreme low and high blood glucose levels and managing the exhaustion that comes with it!

Life once again settled into what I can only describe as a waiting phase.

Having benefited from one of the programs sponsored by JDRF, I became passionate about helping raise funds and awareness about this foundation and its cause. In 2012 JDRF became the charity of choice for the Clipsal 500, the first event for the V8 Supercars season and the biggest for South Australia. Requiring significant input from volunteers to raise awareness and collect donations, I agreed to be at the racing track for the four days to help in whatever capacity was required. This included dressing in the Jelly Baby mascot costume and walking around the grounds (with minders) having photos taken to raise awareness of type 1 diabetes.

There is much confusion about type 1 diabetes. This is further complicated by the fact that when a low blood glucose level occurs, an individual requires some form of quick acting carbohydrate, often in the form of lollies. This is the reason the Jelly Baby is the mascot for JDRF; to promote awareness of the treatment of hypoglycaemia.

However not understanding this can result in confusion and mixed messages.

The Clipsal 500 in 2012 was an opportunity to promote awareness and raise much needed funds for research for that elusive cure. On Thursday March 1st 2012 dressed as a Jelly Baby (and armed with two minders so that I would not trip over or get lost with the limited vision the suit provided) I set out for one last walk around the grounds for photos and last minute donations for the day.

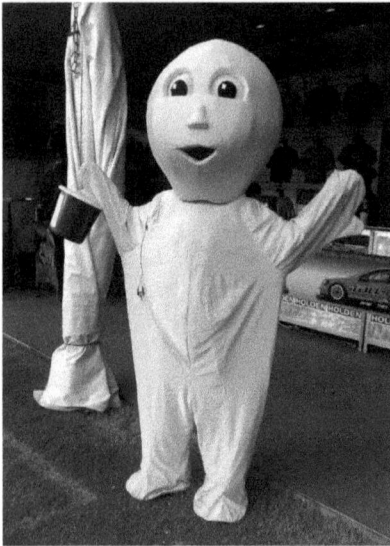

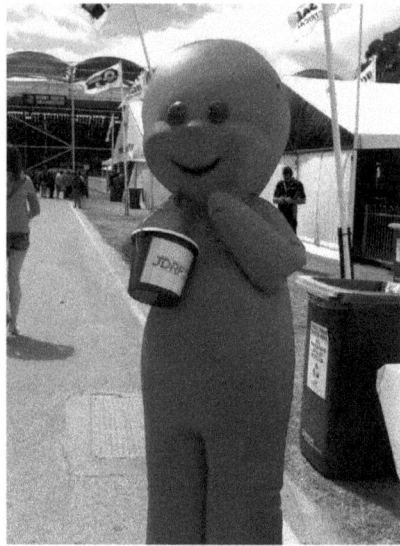

A "deflated" (left) and an "inflated" (right) Jelly Baby raising funds and awareness about type 1 diabetes at Clipsal 500 March 2012

It is difficult to imagine any one person deliberately setting out to intentionally hurt another individual, whether that is by physical or emotional means. However, that is exactly what an individual at Clipsal 500 on 1st March 2012. Having consumed a significant amount of alcohol, presumably throughout the day in a corporate box where his ticket to the four-day event allowed full access, this person decided it would be a good idea to crash-tackle the Jelly Baby mascot! Admittedly the mascot suits require the wearer to be fitted with an air pump to allow the suit to be filled with air and therefore look plump and engaging. They also however require the wearer to be small in stature. This combination is dangerous however when being crash-tackled by someone twice to three times your size, having consumed a considerable amount of alcohol! The result of this inter-action was not favourable to the smaller of the two persons.

Having posed with a small child for photos not moments before, I had turned to continue walking through the crowd of spectators that were mingling awaiting the after-race concert. The next thing I knew (and later recalled) was the smell of alcohol and the feeling of arms wrapped around me and my arms pinned to my side.

I woke up on the cold grass looking at the Jelly Baby's head some metres away (the head of the mascot suit I was wearing that day was separate to the rest of the suit)! While dazed and confused, I attempted to get up before someone told me to lie back down. The one to two hours following this are very hazy with respect to my recollections of the event.

What I do recall is having plenty of support and members of the JDRF team (particularly Tamara and Paul) explaining constantly what was going on and continuing to talk and reassure me.

Unfortunately, due to the nature of my injuries (witnesses to the event say that I landed on my head when I was tackled), there was a question of neck and back complications. For this reason, I required a neck brace, a spinal board and was taken to hospital via ambulance once the Jelly Baby suit was removed!

After approximately seven hours, many scans and some poking and prodding I was thankfully cleared of spinal injuries and sent on my way from the emergency department, albeit without any shoes (you cannot wear shoes in the mascot suit) at approximately 1am.

Again, grateful to not have lasting injuries, it is the support of my dear friends who organised a taxi back to their house, a hot meal when I arrived and a bed to collapse into to that I remember most from the day's events.

While the emergency doctor had warned me that I would be incredibly sore and feel like someone who has whiplash injuries, I wanted to continue to help at the Clipsal 500. All things considered, with the help of Bikram yoga, the overall soreness to my neck, back, arms and right hip (I was hit from behind on the right) settled reasonably quickly and, although traumatised, I tried to not let this event overshadow the success of the four-day opportunity we were given to raise awareness and funds for type 1 diabetes.

However, the long-term recovery from my injuries unfortunately was not to be so simple. Some weeks later, I woke up having had a restless sleep. Swinging my legs out of bed, my right foot felt numb and had pins and needles. My initial (and probably most individuals with diabetes greatest fear) was that this was another complication. Putting my weight on both feet, my right leg did not want to support me! And it did just not feel right.

And so, began my next health journey. For the next two and a half years, I juggled physiotherapists, chiropractors, doctors, remedial massage therapists, orthopaedic surgeons and a sport and exercise medicine physician. I had ultrasounds, CT scans, MRI scans, acupuncture, and two corticosteroid injections in my hip that required a two to three day stay in the critical care unit of a hospital to manage my glucose levels at the same time. (Steroids will cause glucose levels to become elevated but in my case, they become outrageously so for me, and I require management with IV insulin).

The cause of the numbness and pins and needles in my foot? The impact of the crash-tackle had destabilised the ball-and-socket joint in my hip which caused the muscles around this to try to prevent further destabilisation. Unfortunately, over time these muscles became fatigued, causing the symptoms I was experiencing including significant pain in my hip and lower back. The solution? An intense program of exercises to restabilise the ball-and-socket joint. And therapy for pain relief while this occurred!

Managing this, and type 1 diabetes, and holding down a full-time job, was not easy! However, that was what needed to occur. Taking time off work for appointments, and averaging two specialists a week, whether that be allied health or medical, was an expensive exercise! Reducing my working hours through this process was simply not an option. I was told it would take two years of intense rehabilitation, and even then, there was no guarantee that my hip would ever fully return to the same function as before the injury, especially from a pain perspective.

Once again however I am thankful that while the injuries I have sustained are life long, they are manageable, and I am surrounded by amazing, supportive, and wonderful friends and family that continue alongside me through my health journey.

CHAPTER 15

Autoimmunity Anyone?

It is often difficult to negotiate the health care system when you have a chronic health condition. This is especially true for someone with diabetes. Often any symptom, whether caused by diabetes or not, gets blamed on the condition. This has been true a considerable number of times during my life, and an experience shared by many others both with type 1 and type 2 diabetes.

It is unfortunate then that while I had come to accept and manage my pain in my right hip from the Clipsal injury, over time, my hip seemed to be deteriorating and the pain here and, in fact, all over my body, appeared to be getting gradually worse.

More and more I found it difficult to sit for long periods, get in and out of my car and while it seems inconsequential, I became more reluctant to wear high heels because it means the pain in my both hips and lower back the next day was almost unbearable. However, despite numerous conversations with my then GP, blood tests and some scans, I had nothing significant to show for it.

It was not until the pain and symptoms that I had in my right hip began in earnest in my left hip, that I began to really question if there was something more to my pain and severe fatigue that had yet to be discovered. After all, it is certainly not "normal" to have to swap hands at the petrol bowser three to four times while filling up one tank of fuel due to muscle aches, cramping and severe fatigue in your hands and arms. Surely this was not diabetes related even though I had been diagnosed close to forty years ago.

I felt like I constantly had influenza. Not a head cold but actual influenza. My muscles ached all over, I was sore and stiff in the morning and while I felt good for 24 hours after my yoga classes, most forms of exercise were now an extreme struggle, with severe pain a limiting factor of how far and how much I could do.

While working full time with any chronic health condition is difficult, I was still extremely thankful that I had a job I was not only passionate about, but I also loved. While extremely fatigued and finding most days now a juggle with both maintaining healthy glucose levels and managing pain (with absolutely no answers) my sanctuary was helping others. Educating and empowering others in their diabetes journey made me focus on something other than my own health concerns and gave me a sense of purpose each day.

I am a great believer in knowledge. The body is built on a very sophisticated, dynamic equilibrium which we have some knowledge about, but we still have lots to learn. I am fortunate to continue to learn and expand my knowledge, both as a health care professional and as an individual with chronic health needs.

At the time of writing, there was much debate about gluten and its consumption. I was however fortunate enough to be able to have the opportunity to attend a symposium with Alessio Fasano as one of the guest speakers about gluten and its effects on the body. I have always known that, to maintain the lowest fluctuations in my blood glucose levels, an eating plan low in carbohydrates was the best option for me. What I had never considered was that it may not have been the carbohydrates that were impacting but the gluten in these carbo-hydrates that were having the biggest effect on my diabetes.

It is well established that individuals diagnosed with type 1 diabetes are more inclined to develop other forms of autoimmune health conditions, including coeliac disease. I had often been checked for coeliac disease but had always been negative. What I had never been checked for however is the coeliac gene (which is commonly referred to as the risk of developing coeliac disease). What I learned from Dr. Fasano has now changed the management of both my diabetes and my chronic pain.

Gluten is a combination of proteins and used commercially for its bulk and elastic properties. It is found in wheat, rye, barley and can be transported on oat, and other such products as spelt and malt. When added to flour, it improves bread's stability and makes loaves much less crumbly. It is also added to foods as a stabiliser (such as ice cream) and in many sauces and processed meats (such as ham and bacon). When I started investigating what gluten was added to, I was utterly amazed at just how much and what foods (and drinks) it was in!

While there is a difference between coeliac disease and gluten intolerance, both have a huge impact on the body and its ability to function. It is not my intention to persuade any individual to eat a gluten free diet. Rather, again, it is to describe my journey to understanding how to better manage my health conditions and why I have made the decisions I have. Dr Fasano describes "gluten ingestion as a spectrum". Some individuals are not able to tolerate gluten at all (those with coeliac disease), some can eat gluten with no reaction whatsoever, and there are those in the middle or "the murky area of gluten reactions, including gluten sensitivity".

Dr Fasano and a team of researchers at the University of Maryland were able to identify a direct cause between gluten and leaky gut syndrome. What has been shown is that behind the wall of the stomach is something called Gastro Associated Lymphoid Tissue (GALT).

GALT, due to the current lifestyles we all lead can become inundated with toxins, food, and bacteria. It has now been recognised that approximately 80% of the immune system is in the GALT which, when exposed to an onslaught of bacteria and toxins as we eat can become inflamed and damaged. Over time, other systems and organs in the body can also be affected. Known as leaky gut syndrome, this leads to further inflammation and as the gut continues to allow more bacteria and toxins into the body (through holes in the gut wall) this can present as health conditions, including inflammatory and auto-immune disorders. The issue we as a society have, is that gluten has also been identified as a contributor to leaky gut syndrome. Modern day gluten carries pesticides used to kill insects on our crops and causes exposure to the healthy bacteria in our gut. Those individuals more susceptible to health conditions will then begin to develop lowered immune systems due to the breakdown of the GALT and healthy bacteria.

And so, armed with this new information about gluten and its possible effects on my body, I decided to try a gluten free diet. Not because it was trendy, not because it was the "in" thing to do, but because I thought it might be helpful for my diabetes and my pain. I had researched this and there did seem to be credible evidence behind it. It seemed to make sense to trial it for a couple of months and determine the outcome for my well being.

The results? Quite noteworthy. For my diabetes. I am now able to eat more carbohydrates without having such extreme fluctuations in blood glucose levels two hours after food. I now eat more carbohydrates (gluten free of course!) than I have ever eaten but without having to worry as much about what they are going to do to my blood glucose levels two or three hours later. The fluctuations in glucose levels are still there each and every day, as are the hypoglycaemic episodes.

However, I find that I am better able to manage them without having to follow a strict low carbohydrate diet.

While I will not speculate on the mechanism behind what is driving gluten to cause an elevation in my blood glucose levels and the extreme daily fluctuations which I have struggled with the entire time I have been diagnosed with type 1 diabetes my experience indicates that there appears to be a connection for me.

Having followed a gluten free diet as strictly as I possibly can (sometimes accidental exposure can occur when I eat out) for many years, my HbA1c is the lowest it has ever been. Not only this but, my fluctuations in daily glucose levels are of less concern for me, my carbohydrate consumption from day to day is wide and varied and certainly much greater than it has been in the past and my severe hypoglycaemic episodes have also reduced in number. Wanting to explore this further at the outset (I am always one to question the why of things) I asked my then GP if I was able to be gene tested for coeliac disease. Again, I find it remarkably interesting the answers I get from most health care professionals who choose not to practice person centred care (or as I like to refer to it personalised care).

According to the Coeliac Society of Australia, to get a diagnosis of coeliac disease, there must be symptoms of gluten allergy (these are more often than not gut symptoms including diarrhoea, cramping, nausea, vomiting and constipation but can also include skin rashes and joint aches and pains). A diagnosis _**must**_ occur after a stomach biopsy that shows changes to the lining of intestine. I did not show the "typical signs" of gluten allergy. I did not have the stomach symptoms. Nor did I show the "typical signs of damage" to my gastrointestinal lining indicative with a stomach biopsy. I did however have a rash, something I had put up with since my second transplant and something that no health care professional had been able to explain except to label as "dermatitis". However, dermatitis herpetiformis is a rash of which I had all the symptoms, and it is associated with coeliac disease.

Dermatitis herpetiformis is a rash that often presents as blisters filled with watery fluid (I first noticed these blisters years ago on my heels of my feet in the same spots on each foot). The age of onset is usually between 15-40 (but can affect both young and old) and once again although the exact cause is not known, it has been linked to coeliac disease.

Interestingly dermatitis herpetiformis was first described in 1884 by Louis Aldophus During and is not any way linked to the herpes virus. It is however associated with the HLA-DQ2 haplotype.

A haplotype is a physical grouping of variants that residue closely together on a chromosome and tend to be inherited together. The basis behind studying haplotypes is to extract information and aid investigations in localising disease-causing genes.

My rash appeared to be significantly worse when gluten was ingested.

Signs of dermatitis herpetiformis include intense, itchy, chronic eruptions that are often unbearable and look like red bumps or blisters. While they often occur at the back of the neck, scalp, elbows, knees, hairline, groin, or face, mine thankfully were mostly confined to the scalp and occasionally to my hairline and fingers. However, despite enormous discomfort and the rash often causing pain and extreme itching and burning, I had never had any of gastrointestinal symptoms so common in those that have coeliac disease! Once again this was never mentioned to me nor was dermatitis herpetiformis ever offered as a possible explanation to a condition that plagued me for years!

Each year, to maintain my professional qualifications I am required to update my knowledge. I had stumbled upon this ailment when reading about other dermatological conditions for my home medication review exams. I found myself once more needing to "plead my case" as to why I wanted to have gene testing for coeliac disease. What I found most interesting again through all my discussions was the need to consistently ask for investigations to be carried out. While I acknowledge there is the capacity for some individuals to need extra attention without any real health conditions, I am not one of these and I had actual rashes with blisters that were evident almost all the time. I did eventually get the gene testing for coeliac disease done however and the results came back positive on both the HLA-DQ2 and HLA-DQ8 gene. This meant I had a high risk of developing coeliac disease at some point in my life.

Again, what I found interesting is the lack of understanding of coeliac disease, gluten, and some health professionals' reaction to questions about this. According to Dr Fasano, for many years now the health industry has believed "you have coeliac disease or nothing else". However, as an expert in this field, he believes that there is significant evidence that, if genetically predisposed, gluten can be a harmful toxin and the body will mount different responses in different individuals. Such responses include joint pain, inflammation, foggy brain, anaemia, miscarriages, infertility, rashes, chronic headache, and schizophrenia! From the time I listened to Dr Fasano speak at the conference, I have remained strictly gluten free (more than 10 years at the time of first publishing this book) and in that time my fluctuations in glucose levels from day to day were much lower and the rash that had plagued me for almost ten years was almost non-existent (except when I accidentally got exposed when eating out)! I had not been given, at the time of writing this chapter, any formal diagnosis of what was causing my rash but if eating gluten free is a way of managing the symptoms then again this is what I am prepared to do!

While it is interesting that I have had to draw my own conclusions from my research, this is not uncommon in many health conditions. What is remarkably interesting is the number of opposing opinions I have had from health care professionals about my new choice of eating gluten free! To this I have responded on two levels:

1. If the health care professional is not prepared to engage in personalised care, then they shall not be included as part of my health care team.
2. Gluten free has helped me significantly manage my diabetes and that is a reason for me to remain eating this way.

Did I have dermatitis herpetiformis? I was not 100% convinced that this was the exact cause of my blisters in my scalp because they continued to appear even when I knew I had not been exposed to gluten for long periods of time. What I did know was the rash seemed worse when I was exposed and there was no health care professional that could give me a logical explanation for it.

Unfortunately, however the gluten free option did not have the same overwhelming positive impact on my pain as it did on my diabetes. In fact, if anything my pain appeared to be getting worse and had moved to more muscles and joints. Without any real indication of where to refer next, I was sent to a pain specialist.

Pain is very subjective. There is no "test" that can accurately describe to a medical professional the degree of pain, or what type of pain an individual is experiencing. Pain is also multifaceted and can change from day to day and within a day, depending on other influences such as mood and, for me, blood glucose levels. So, to describe to a stranger, albeit, well-educated and highly experienced, the nature and type of pain that I had been experiencing with increasing intensity for now what seemed like an eternity, but in actual time was approximately four years, was difficult. Nonetheless I tried my best.

The response? My diabetes. Or more to the point, I was "burnt out because of my chronic health condition" (insert diabetes) and that appeared to be "manifesting in physical symptoms". Oh, and I was "depressed"!

While not one to easily self reflect, I will admit at this point I was prepared to consider any suggestion. There are always days and times when any chronic health condition, regardless of which one it is, can be difficult. Diabetes is certainly no different. And I am no different. However, upon reflection, and knowing what I know about burn out, this did not seem relevant to my symptoms. Diabetes burnout is often described as a disregard for blood glucose levels and forgetting to take insulin. The psychological symptoms include stress, anxiety, depression, anger, resentment, shame, and guilt. Having certainly experienced these and diabetes burnout in my late twenties, I knew this was not the same. Although fatigue could certainly be associated with these, I am not inclined to believe intense overwhelming, unforgiving pain is!

And so once again I am so thankful to my parents who gave me the confidence to be able to express my opinion respectfully but forcefully. I oversee my health and I am very much entitled to an opinion when it comes to this. While the pain specialist had his diagnosis, I respectfully informed him that I did not agree that I was either burnt out or depressed having to live with a chronic health condition. I had days when I found it more difficult than others, and this did have an impact on my mental health, but it was not the reason for my overwhelming pain. And while the pain specialist's words told me I "was certainly entitled to have an opinion", his body language informed me quite differently. And so, I was back to the drawing board with what to do and where to go.

Fortunately, by this time, I had started to build a health care team that I was not only comfortable with, but who were prepared to listen and consider my opinion. Enter another "ologist" in the form of a rheumatologist.

Having a strong family history of rheumatoid arthritis, and an autoimmune condition already in the form of type 1 diabetes, the logical referral for the type of pain I was experiencing was to a physician who specialised in musculoskeletal disease. Given the fact that I had asked for this referral and felt once again I needed to "plead my case" to my then GP, I felt it was time to change to someone whom I felt would practise personalised care. Enter new GP and rheumatologist who I must say at this point I am incredibly grateful for and extremely pleased to have found!

While at first, I felt that I was going to end up with a similar diagnosis to that which I had been given by the pain specialist (chronic pain syndrome from lack of sleep due to the continuous glucose monitor breaking my cycle of sleep over and over) here was someone who (like many of the members of the rest of my team) practiced individualised care. Having sent me away for numerous tests (blood tests and scans and a corticosteroid injection into my right hip meaning ANOTHER two-night stay in hospital for diabetes management) to determine if this helped with the pain, I felt like my pain, fatigue, and soreness were being taken seriously. The result? Nothing on blood tests, and unfortunately the corticosteroid did not make my pain any better (although the two-day bed rest made my hip pain better but my lower back pain worse). However, MRI scans found something-finally!

As much as I did not want to have another autoimmune disease, I did want to have a diagnosis so I could get on with it! Drum roll please… After almost six years of complaining of pain and fatigue… Spondylarthritis, an arthritis which affects the joints of the spine, pelvis, shoulders, and hips. It can also affect the areas where the ligaments and tendons attach to the bones. While in most cases spondylarthritis attacks the spine, it can also affect the hands, feet, arms, and legs. This explains why I was in so much pain and felt fatigued most of the time. There is a strong genetic component to the development of spondylarthritis and, interestingly from the research I have since done there are scientists that also believe it may be caused from a bacterium entering the bowel (the gluten and leaky gut theory).

So once again the problem for me was that my body did not "follow the rules". My spondylarthritis is what is known as seronegative arthritis which means that it does not show on blood tests. The inflammatory markers that health professionals look for to diagnose and determine what medicines to give did not show up in my blood. Where did that leave me? Struggling for six years to plead my case that I wasn't "depressed", that it wasn't my "diabetes", and it wasn't "burn out" causing my symptoms. It also now left me once again "negotiating" with the health care system to get treatment for my arthritis. You see the PBS (Pharmaceutical Benefits Scheme) has a list of medicines for each health condition and criteria that you must match to be prescribed each and every medicine. Because I did not have any markers in my blood that "indicated" I had auto-immune arthritis I had to stick to the medicines that did not agree with me and were much less effective. But at this point I was prepared to try anything.

And so, we began to explore the medicines that may (or may not) help with reducing my body attacking its own joints.

Methotrexate comes with a long list of nasty side effects. If used in high doses it is an anti-cancer medicine. However, if used in low doses it is used to suppress the immune system and helps alleviate pain, inflammation and swelling in joints. It can unfortunately cause nausea, vomiting and diarrhoea, all things that can destabilise type 1 diabetes. Oh, the joy of now managing more than one chronic health condition! My first dose was injected cautiously at the GP's rooms with the endocrinologist on standby in case I needed to go to hospital. However, none of the side effects that were listed in the literature were a problem for me at all! And the benefits of pain relief and reduction in swelling were almost immediate! Within twelve hours I noticed my pain score reduce from 8/10 to 5/10! I do not think I had realised just how sore I was until I had started taking the methotrexate. What a difference it made!

And so, began the weekly injections of methotrexate. Every Monday morning, I injected it to help reduce the symptoms of my arthritis. And I took folic acid to offset the gastrointestinal symptoms (nausea, vomiting and diarrhoea of which so far, I had experienced none). Unfortunately, however the methotrexate was not enough to stop the destruction of my joints and the all the pain. And over time what became more obvious was that while my initial symptoms fitted with spondylarthritis, it was looking more like I had rheumatoid arthritis instead.

Rheumatoid arthritis causes pain and inflammation in the joints (places where the bones meet). Although common in the hands, knees, and feet it is also affects eyes and lungs. Over time, while I had pain in all the areas mentioned, I was noticing more and more that mornings were becoming difficult for me to move, and I was unable to walk properly especially if I had been standing on my feet all day at work. My diagnosis was changed to rheumatoid, and we again tried many combinations of medicines with the methotrexate to see if we could get my pain score lower than 5/10.

The complication once again was both my diabetes and that of not having markers in my blood indicating that I had arthritis. All but one of all the other classes of medicines used to treat rheumatoid arthritis are either not able to be used due to my other health

conditions or I had tried and had extreme side effects, including suicidal tendencies and problems with my heart! This made it exceedingly difficult when there was constant swapping and changing of
medicines without any quantifying arthritis markers.

Having trialled and failed with all the medicines available the
only option left was to apply for special access for medicines known
as the TNF inhibitors. These medicines were awfully expensive under
the PBS so those who have rheumatoid arthritis need to qualify with
arthritis blood markers before the government will pay for them to be
written on an authority prescription. I did not qualify (seronegative
arthritis) and I had run out of all other options to treat my pain and
stiffness, my rheumatologist made an application for special circumstances. What should have taken a couple of weeks took three months.
However finally (and after nearly not being able to work from pain
and fatigue despite the methotrexate initially being amazingly effective) I started my first injection (these injections were fortnightly)
with amazing results! Within twelve hours my pain score had dropped
again. This time to a 2.5/10. As well as the pain dropping, my fatigue
reduced significantly, my fingers no longer hurt (and they no longer
felt like sausages) and I did not feel like I constantly had influenza! I
was no longer sore and stiff when I got up in the mornings and now,
I did not look at Tupperware and taps with dread! Those of you with
any form of arthritis will understand this last statement about how
tricky turning taps on and off are! And Tupperware lids are a whole
other level of challenging concept that is more difficult to solve than
a Rubik's cube! Now, after only two injections two weeks apart, I was
able to enjoy Bikram yoga again and did not feel like I had been hit
by a bus both while I practised yoga and for two to three days after
I had finished.

With the methotrexate self-injected every Monday morning and
the new medicine injected every two weeks on a Friday, I felt I was

able to adequately manage both my diabetes and my auto-immune arthritis and felt that life was getting back on track after more than six years of uncertainty.

But yes, you are right.

I spoke too soon!

One Thursday morning when I woke up, swung my feet out of bed to the side of the floor, went to stand up and felt like I had broken almost every bone in both my feet! This was approximately three months into the start of my new methotrexate/TNF inhibitor regimen when all was going well, and I was feeling great (apart from the odd twinge from my hips and other joints).

After a very slow start to the morning (the shower was a long one to entice my feet to understand they were not "allowed" to spend the day in bed and actually had to cooperate at some point in that morning) I managed to make my way to work and put a call into my rheumatologist. Throughout the day my feet did seem to cooperate and the pain dulled somewhat so by the time he returned my call, I did begin to wonder if it was simply morning stiffness I was experiencing from a flare. (A flare is a term often use to describe a period of increased disease activity usually recognised by a worsening of symptoms). Having had reasonable success from the medications and not yet knowing what would cause an increase in an inflammatory response for me, I was yet to know when I would have a flare and what would cause it (if I was even able to identify such triggers).

Despite feeling some relief by the end of the day, I was called back to the specialist's office the following Monday for another round of many tests including checking for gout and my liver and kidney health. While the medicines are fantastic at "dumbing down" my immune system, they come with side effects and unfortunately these are wide and can be toxic if not monitored carefully. Suddenly after three months of limited or no side effects, my liver enzymes had become extremely elevated! So much so that I had to stop the methotrexate immediately because it seemed that it was the most likely culprit to cause this to occur. However, this was not what had caused my feet to feel like I had broken all the bones in them. This was something entirely different. My rheumatologist had also run a check for systemic lupus erythematosus (lupus) and this had come back positive! This test was checking for antibodies to ds-DNA (double stranded DNA). While often this can be drug induced, it also did fit with my symptoms that I had before injecting TNF inhibitors. When antibodies are present for ds-DNA (with symptoms) it is almost always conclusive for the diagnosis of lupus!

Medicine can be extremely complicated and complex, and I do not begin to pretend I understand most of it at the best of times. However, I am fortunate enough, as I have said earlier, that I was born with both intelligence and an inquisitive mind. I know I was previously tested for lupus and tested negative so when I was given this news I was not overly concerned about the diagnosis because some TNF inhibitors can cause this to occur and stopping it will prevent further problems (again a well-known side effect and called drug induced lupus). The problem for me now was I had to cease both the methotrexate (due to my liver enzymes being so elevated and give it time to recover) AND the TNF inhibitor. SO, I was back to where I had been for the last six years, in pain, very fatigued and with no solutions for pain management for at least one month, or thereabouts the specialist told me! And a festive season to get through! Not to mention the worry about what if I had lupus?

CHAPTER 16

From Someone Else's Perspective

I thought it appropriate to ask one of my very dear friends to write a chapter on their perspective of my life and health conditions. Tam, I believe has a very real awareness of life with diabetes and I am touched by her words.

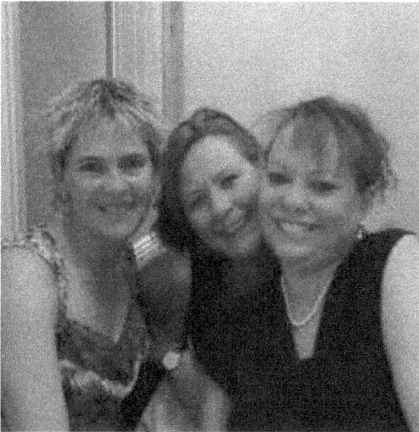

Paul and Tam's 1 yr. Anniversary

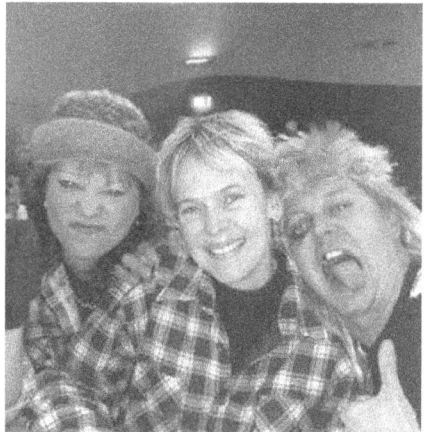

A Bogan Bingo Fundraiser

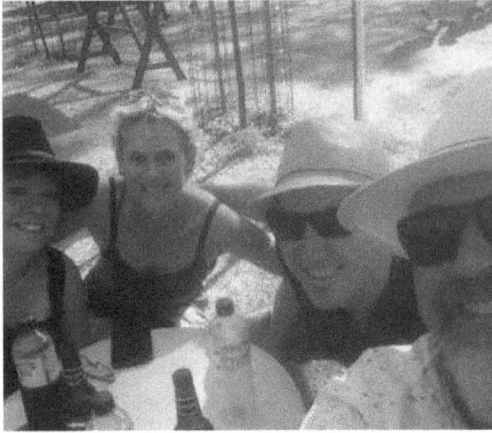

Great times at the Fringe

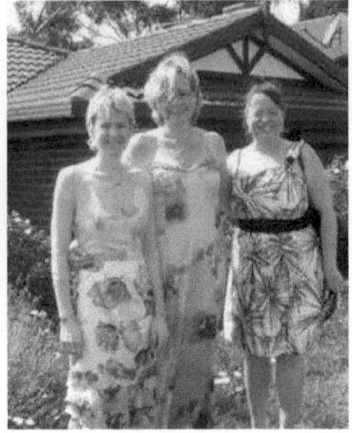

Heading off to
Tam's Hens Day

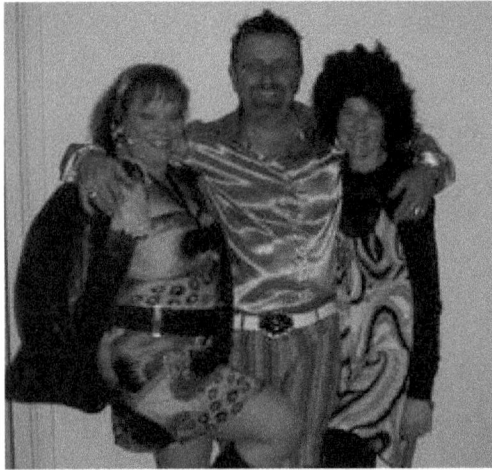

At a mutual friend's 30th birthday

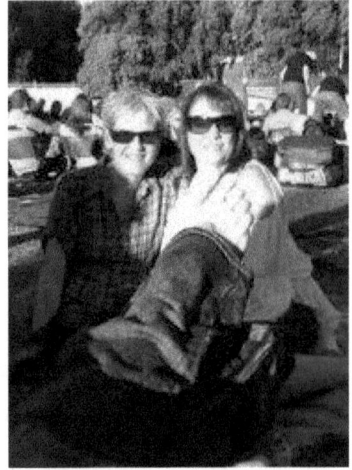

A birthday for Tam at
Botanic Park Cinema

I was very fortunate to begin my role as Development Manager for JDRF in SA on February 6th, 2006. Not knowing extensive amounts about type 1 diabetes nor the SA landscape for the role I had just embarked on, I was very fortunate to meet a band of dedicated fundraisers in the lead up to their Golf Event held at the Mt Barker Golf Club very early in my role. From the outset Kirrily was the standout event organiser of this event and soon became the person I would liaise with throughout. Having lived in the Mt Barker region for many years this was Kirrily's backyard and the golf event, its participation and fundraising from raffle and auction was hugely successful.

Funds raised from the Golf Event supported Kirrily and her team including Alex and Jan, for their entry into the JDRF Barossa One Ride, an event that began in 2004 and concluded in 2018. This dedicated trio were always present, rode their hearts out and became widely recognised at the event. In the later years of the event and a result of Kirrily's changing health needs it was great to see the event was possible with some E Bikes. And even when Kirrily could not ride this did not stop her participating and supporting the event in a fundraising capacity.

It was my absolute pleasure to support Kirrily's many years of fundraising when she required and to get to spend the weekend with her in the Barossa, once per year in January. Awarded a yellow jersey for 3 years, a Foundation Cycling Club Jersey for 4 years, a plaque at year 5 and a special recognition jersey at year ten, it was my greatest pleasure to nominate Kirrily for the 2009 Leanne Chronican Spirit Award – for teamwork, commitment to fundraising, and a can-do attitude. This prestigious award, given to very few of the 300 or more cyclists per year, was enthusiastically supported by the crowd's cheers and applause.

But this was not the only award I bestowed on Kirrily, nominating her for the 2008 State Volunteer of the Year - for event support, fundraising support, guest speaking and mentorship and for her part in on the SA Ride to Cure Diabetes Committee in 2013, including the award the Committee received as State Volunteers of the Year.

Our now 15-year friendship that was born through my work commitment and Kirrily's own type 1 diabetes journey from her childhood has encompassed many business-related and personal events and gatherings. Kirrily has supported many JDRF fundraising activities, events, and family gatherings. She continues to support JDRF's mission – to accelerate life-changing breakthroughs to cure, treat and prevent type 1 diabetes.

Kirrily's roles have been many and varied including supporting JDRF as a guest speaker at Parliament House, JDRF breakfasts and networking events and more recently with her business colleague Jayne Lehmann as a guest speaker at the Virtual JDRF Summit in 2021. This earned her and Jayne "best presenter" status for the event. I appreciated their honesty as they themselves navigate their own journey with type 1 diabetes.

As a dedicated advocate and Credentialled Diabetes Educator Kirrily is passionate about raising awareness, correcting misconceptions about type 1 and type 2 diabetes, and ensuring those living with type 1 diabetes have a voice, ensuring the health system that supports them is doing just that. Never one to judge, having lived with type 1 diabetes for most of her life, I value Kirrily's support of those I refer to her and direction provided for those in need. Kirrily is a wonderful role model for all other diabetes education staff. She is thorough, considerate and a wealth of knowledge. In 2016 Kirrily was awarded ADEA (Australian Diabetes Educator Association) CDE of the year in SA then went on to be recognised by her peers and was a dual winner (with Ann Morris) of the National Award the same year. So well deserved for someone who gives so much.

I have listened in awe when Kirrily has spoken about type 1 diabetes and support. Her no holds barred approach ensures she gets her message across. There is never any grey with Kirrily. It's all black and white. I have listened as she has spoken with me of her own type 1 diabetes journey, her islet cell transplants, the success and the challenges of this explorative treatment, the scarring, the heart ache, the recovery, the back to the drawing board. By listening to Kirrily I am sure it has made me more aware, more thoughtful, more supportive of those who live with this chronic auto-immune condition that is type 1 diabetes and makes me even more determined to keep working with JDRF to find a cure, better treatments, and prevention for those yet diagnosed.

Now to a slightly more personal note of a friendship that began in early 2006 and has been unwavering since and will extend beyond my work if I was ever to depart JDRF.

Married to my husband Paul in 2011 it was a pleasure to have Kirrily at my hen's day and Paul's and my wedding and then our one-year anniversary at Enzo's restaurant. This gathering was reserved for just a few of our wedding guests. Kirrily and I have celebrated many a birthday together, no doubt always celebrating way too much! From your everyday birthdays to significant 40th birthdays for us both and my husband and my 50th Birthday in 2021 we have always made the time to come together. With the Adelaide Fringe close to Kirrily's birthday it always provided another reason to enjoy some comedy at the Fringe and festival food and drink. I look forward to celebrating Kirrily's half century with her in 2023.

I am equally grateful to have been asked to support my dear friend at her father Des's funeral, something I hold very dear. Covid had restricted numbers of who could attend so I was pleased I could be there in Kirrily's time of need when many others were restricted from attending.

But as a friend we are tied together more than just the years of friendship or JDRF or type 1 diabetes. Both dog lovers, adorers, and absolute nuts for our fur babies we have been through heartache together at the loss of beautiful Banjo, Bailey, and Cooper. Whilst nothing will ever replace our love for our lost puppies, we can now enjoy our new loves in Koda and Marley and hopefully one day they will soon meet.

Here's to many more years of friendship Kirrily. Thank you for inviting me into your world.

CHAPTER 17

Systemic Lupus Erythematosus

There are many different types of lupus but the most common is systemic lupus erythematosus. Once again, this health condition is due to a faulty immune system attacking the body. Symptoms are determined by what parts of the body are targeted but include:

- skin rashes (both on the face and body)

- **joint and muscle pain**

- hair loss

- **fatigue**

- **fever**

- **headaches/migraines**

- **confusion and memory problems**

- **anxiety** and depression

- **mouth** and nose ulcers

- blood and blood vessel problems, such as high blood pressure, **anaemia, and increased risk of blood clots**

- chest pain and/or breathlessness (because of inflammation of the lining of the heart or lungs)

- poor kidney function-if the immune system attacks the kidneys

- seizures or visual disturbances (a rare symptom resulting from inflammation of the nervous system)

- abdomen pain (a less frequent symptom caused by inflammation of the gut, pancreas, liver, or spleen).

Among the list of symptoms above, the ailments that I had been continually and constantly experiencing and reporting back to the health care professionals (only to be told mostly that there was "nothing remarkable in my bloods") I have highlighted in dark ink. And once again from the many hours of research I have done my understanding is that lupus is a difficult autoimmune condition to diagnose due but not exclusively to the fact there is no definitive test. There are greatly varying symptoms (depending on which organs are affected) and it can often mimic other health conditions! Lupus can also take months if not years to arrive at a diagnosis point! All of this was now ringing true for me!

And so, the complexity of the autoimmune cascade had now become even more dense! No longer did I have a diagnosis of sero-negative arthritis, supposedly! Instead, I now had a diagnosis of systemic lupus erythematosus.

"Systemic" means the whole system as opposed to only one part, "lupus" means inflammation of the skin, and "erythematosus" is from the Greek word erythros, or red, which refers to the reddish colour of the circular shaped facial rash that is distinctive for most individuals who get lupus.

This rash however was not present with my lupus, again making the diagnosis so much harder. Continuing with the theme of my health history, my antibodies to ds-DNA did not disappear once I ceased the TNF inhibitor and no matter how long I waited they did not reduce in number. This is what we were hoping because it would have been a diagnosis of "drug induced lupus". Over the months the titre (or number) of antibodies increased in my blood. And so, I was given the official diagnosis! Not drug-induced but actual lupus!

Was I frustrated with the length of time it took for yet another diagnosis? ABSOLUTELY! Did this mean that we were back to ground zero for medications because generally TNF inhibitors are not shown to be overly effective in lupus? Yes! But what again I struggled with most was the concept of personalised care! Again, I continued to stress to my specialist that I struggled each and EVERY day to get out of bed and perform basic duties! Putting a key in the front door, filling my car up with petrol, getting things out of my handbag (my knuckles of my hands were just too sore), holding a pen, walking more than 100 metres, turning on taps, gardening, housework, shopping, sitting, or standing for more than one hour at a time. And yet he continued to tell me that it was NOT the lupus causing this!! This statement confused me on several levels:

1. Does not all literature state that lupus can cause joint and muscle pain??
2. If it was not lupus causing this, then was it something else that had been missed?

I again started doing my own research as this seemed the logical step for me given the history behind the prolonged diagnosis. As previously stated, when an individual is diagnosed with one autoimmune condition, they are more prone to be diagnosed with another. So, two (or three) could potentially increase the likelihood of a fourth. Such as rheumatoid arthritis? And such a thing exists and is given the nickname "rupus". Again, when questioned the answer I got was a simple "no". With no explanation and no discussion entered into.

Having had a minimum of three months of no medication (to allow my liver time to recover from the other medicine) where I simply had no pain relief and had to spend every moment when I was not at work resting, I was finally able to recommence methotrexate injections because my liver enzymes had begun to settle back into the healthy range. However, my pain levels were still greatly elevated and day to day living was extremely compromised. Again, the search began for a reasonable medicine that would allow for positive impact without major side effects. Unfortunately, once again the side effects of most of these medicines were too significant to bear!

Two of the most frequently used oral medicines to treat lupus caused mental health issues for me! In fact, one caused severe night panic attacks, chest pain and dry eyes to the point I was unable to see! However, I again had to prove that it was the medicine doing this and not the lupus. Unable to have a reasonable conversation about these side effects, I stopped taking it and then restarted to "prove" my point to both my rheumatologist and ophthalmologist because "it was determined it was highly doubtful this was an unlikely side effect". Once proven (personalised care anyone?) however, a second agent was chosen. This one caused suicidal tendencies and again I had to "plead my case". This time I simply stopped taking them until a solution could be sorted. Again, it is lucky I am not going to ever allow any individual to dictate the conditions of my healthcare and will continue to seek the best possible solution for myself in the current climate. Together my health care team and I were finally able to find a combination of medicines (although not common) that seemed to work for me and keep my ds-DNA titre under control.

Was my pain completely under control? No! Was my lupus titre satisfactory according to my rheumatologist- apparently yes! Again, this is the problem with pain. It is very subjective and there is no way to measure any individual's score nor match one individual's pain threshold against another's. How then do you adequately relate to this as a specialist unless you have experienced overwhelming long-term systemic pain? Could I function each day and hold down a full-time job? Yes! Was I still able to go to Bikram Yoga which was still one of my passions? Yes! But that was pretty much it for me! I worked full time and went to yoga once a week. The rest of my time was spent recovering from these two activities. Was I sore and in pain most days and did this pain change hourly and from day to day? Absolutely! I was unable to determine what made this pain worse or better and which joints were going to be affected any day or any week. It was like Russian Roulette most mornings to determine which joint my body was going to "pick" on any given day. Please do not get me wrong, I do not write this for sympathy or for attention. It is simply to raise the awareness of autoimmune conditions and how each individual sometimes needs to take responsibility for their own health – and that individual was me! The only way I can describe my new normal was my body now felt like the first 24-48 hours after I had run a marathon with little training. I am sure most people have felt that joint and muscle soreness after they have decided to restart exercise after a long break! Those days of muscle soreness following such a rash decision are a killer! For me (and potentially many that live with lupus every day) this had been my reality for several years. Now it had a name and was finally being treated! Systemic lupus erythematosus.

CHAPTER 18

#wearenotwaiting

Through all the issues with pain and changes to my eating patterns and medicine, one of the most difficult things was the constant juggle of my diabetes management. Here were all the extra influences on glucose levels that I had very little control over! An extreme pain day meant an enormous impact on my glucose levels, and that in turn would impact on my pain! I had little or no ability to have much influence over this except to treat accordingly and to move on with my day.

Having the invention of the CGM (continuous glucose monitoring) with its increased accuracy gave me the ability to know not only what my glucose levels were doing at any given minute of the day; it also meant I knew where they had been and where they were going because the system told me via trend arrows. For those that have never used CGM it is a bit like driving a car. Blood glucose monitoring via standard finger pricking is like driving a car down a freeway at 100 kms an hour, opening your eyes every couple of minutes and expecting not to hit anything. CGM is like driving the car with your eyes open and having a GPS!

Over time, changes to my daily exercise routine and the inflammatory response in my body due to potentially more than two autoimmune conditions had not only a detrimental effect on my glucose levels, but also I began to see a greater impact on glucose fluctuations and my HbA1c. If that were even possible!

Again, not one to accept that there was nothing I could do at this point for my own health, I had discovered through online posts there was an emerging new treatment option for people with diabetes that used artificial intelligence to help in the management of type 1 diabetes. I had also discovered it was quite secretive and certainly not FDA (Food and Drug Administration; Federal Agency of the Department of Health and Ageing in America) or TGA (Therapeutic Goods Administration in Australia) approved! However, given my latest diabetes results had come back slightly elevated and I estimated I was dedicating 2-3 hours each day to my health management, I felt any changes I could make at this point might be worth a consideration.

When an individual is wearing sensor augmented therapy (which describes a CGM and an insulin pump) there is a significant amount of reaction required from the person with diabetes. Dana Lewis, one of the individuals behind the Open APS (Artificial Pancreas System) describes this as "constantly responding to fire alarms all the time". Once you have worn CGM for a while there can be a shift to understanding that there can be a combination of proactivity and reactivity in diabetes management. This was my next step in understanding looping (and is known as open looping). Having worn both an insulin pump and CGM for quite some time I wanted to understand how I could begin to use an algorithm to adjust insulin doses (both basal and boluses) based on recommendations made on the glucose levels being constantly fed back through a system. This system is known as an APS or artificial pancreas system and while it has been around for some time is not commonly promoted commercially. When I first saw the APS acronym, I spent hours looking for what it was short for and could not find it anywhere! Obvious right? Did I mention anywhere this is like a secret club??!!

The next step from the open loop system was for me to explore what was known as the closed loop system where instead of recommendations being made by the algorithm and the person acting on these recommendations, the system acts instead without any intervention from the wearer! The change in quality of life and reduction in burden was, from what I had read and understood, immeasurable!

And so, with some trepidation I set about trying to find out as much as I could about the #wearenotwaiting community, the DIY (do it yourself) systems and looping itself. What I stumbled across was the most generous and encouraging group of people I have ever met! These like-minded individuals have one goal in common and that is for everyone to experience the freedom of what people without diabetes take for granted, that is blood glucose levels in range as often as possible with little or no hypoglycaemia and truly little involvement from the individual. Truly little involvement from day to day! To have this amazing advantage you need a CGM (continuous glucose monitor) and an insulin pump that can be controlled by a computer plus a radio transmitter that connects the pump and CGM. Then there is a smartphone that connects all these components together.

After hours of research and talking to people both online and at some face to face meetings I discovered there are two main setups for looping - OpenAPS and Loop, compatible with android and I-Phones respectively. Looping works by collecting information about glucose levels from my continuous monitoring device on my phone App and sharing this information. An algorithm loaded onto another App on my phone then makes the decision to change the insulin basal doses in my pump and communicates this to my pump via Bluetooth. The most exciting thing about this system is the glucose data from the continuous glucose monitor (and therefore uploading and changing of basal rates in my pump via the algorithm) occurs every five minutes.

This whole new way of managing diabetes is not FDA (America) nor TGA (Australia) approved, and the companies that make the insulin pumps are extremely nervous when their insulin pump is used for "off label" purposes. Sourcing a pump that has the capacity to Loop can therefore be quite difficult!

As I have previously indicated there is a significant amount of secrecy surrounding this movement which I believe stems from the fact that diabetes generates a large amount of money for companies making medicine and technology for us to stay alive and well. I am not immune to this money. I make a living both as a pharmacist and a credentialled diabetes educator which may make me a hypocrite and perhaps many will think this after you have read this. This is your opinion, and you are very much entitled to it! Once I stumbled across Looping (and stumbled is the only word I could use to describe how I discovered this new type of management for diabetes), I struggled to come to terms with the fact that there is a divide between who in our society has the capacity to access this technology and who has not. This will become a little clearer later.

DIY clearly "interrupts" the chain of supply of money and forces somewhat uncomfortable conversations around whose responsibility is it if something were to go seriously wrong with insulin delivery. Remember, we are now discussing an algorithm in a computer adjusting insulin doses in an insulin pump based on information it is receiving with no intervention from the individual with diabetes!

Therefore, to Loop I must write my own code or what is known as building my own automated delivery system. This is the algorithm that tells my pump how much to change the basal rate when the glucose level is coming in as information to the pump. The reason for this is really two-fold. The first is so I understand how the loop works. This is a great built in safety mechanism so I can understand how the algorithm comes up with the changes to the basal rate on my insulin pump every five minutes and allows me to be able to fix problems as they occur (as with any technology there can be problems that need to be addressed from time to time). The second and potentially one of the most important points about health and technology comes down once again to responsibility.

Scheduling is a national classification system that controls how medicines and poisons are made available to the public. In Australia, medicines and poisons are classified into Schedules according to the level of regulatory control over the availability of the medicine or poison required to protect public health and safety (www.tga.gov.au/scheduling-basics). At the time of writing this chapter, insulin is classed in Australia as what is known as a schedule 4 item. This means it is a prescription only medicine or prescription animal remedy. Only those who can write prescriptions can make changes to insulin doses unless of course it is the person with diabetes (or in some cases their carer such as a parent in the case of a child).

In the case of Looping where an algorithm can make changes to the doses of insulin for me (whether that is in the form of a bolus or a basal rate) the only person that is able to write the code for this is me, the person with diabetes. Otherwise, there are all sorts of legalities around who made the changes in the insulin doses and who is responsible if something goes wrong with such a change.

And so, while the start-up (and upgrades that occur on a regular basis) was challenging for me to get my head around initially, especially when I was not computer literate, the actual writing of the code that programs the Loop has to be written by me each time. This ensures when the algorithm makes changes to the insulin pump basal rate in theory, the changes are being made by the person with diabetes. And importantly the responsibility of those changes stays with the person with diabetes (or carer). This allowed for the legality of the scheduling of insulin to still be in place with the Looping set up.

Despite the cloak of secrecy, and ups and downs of the delayed diagnosis of Lupus, I was able to start Looping for the management of my diabetes. Was this easy? HELL NO! I had NO clue on how to code or which system was better, or whether I should choose an Android phone over an iPhone! Is it worth it? HELL yes! I am in range so much more than I ever was without looping! For much much much much much less daily effort! And as a bonus recently I had one of the lowest HbA1c results I have ever recorded (even lower than when I was involved with the transplantation process). Is it safe? As far as I am aware, absolutely! As safe as any other system I have ever used, and I have used every type of management available for diabetes (both type 1 and type 2) over the years! Why am I writing about this system when it is so hush hush? There is nothing that I have written about here that is not available on the open Internet for anyone to see! Do I struggle that there are so many individuals that are not aware of looping and will not be able to access for many reasons some as simple as they are simply not able to afford the hardware that is required (insulin pump and CGM)? Absolutely! I struggle that I make my living not necessarily being able to offer this in regular discussion with clients because health care professionals are not covered by their insurance to even have an open discussion because these systems are not approved by regulatory bodies. **I am not endorsing Looping for the management of diabetes.** I am simply telling you my personal story and the success I have had. Has Looping taken the focus off one of my autoimmune conditions? Simply put YES! And it is my decision to weigh the advantages and disadvantages against each other and to make the decision for my own health!

I would also like to acknowledge the wonderful on and off-line support I have had in setting up and maintaining my loop. I have never in all my years of living with diabetes nor finding my way with other autoimmune conditions felt so supported and "normal". This means so much. To those who know who you are THANK YOU x

CHAPTER 19

Rupus It Is Not!

And so as one decade slowly rolled to an end and another loomed before me, I had come to terms with what I believed was the best I could do for my health. I had negotiated what I believed to be the best outcomes based on all the information that I had available to me despite numerous roadblocks along the way. I had discovered management options that I could only term "elite" and while this saddened me, I was also very glad that I, at least, was able to take advantage of these options. By the end of 2019, I felt I had arrived at a place in my health where I was going to be able to maintain status quo and begin to focus on something other than just surviving. Of course, I forgot to consult my body on this which once again had completely different plans!

Despite regular conversations about how sore all my joints and muscles were (both the small and large joints including toes, ankles, knees, hips, fingers, wrists, back, neck, hands and ribs - it often hurt to breathe) and how very fatigued I was most of the time, it was decided by my health team repeatedly that this was simply due to my lupus. However, despite my medicine, I was not getting any better. Again, while I asked about whether I may also have rheumatoid arthritis and was told this was not the case, what was only considered for a fleeting moment was psoriatic arthritis.

Psoriatic Arthritis

Psoriatic arthritis is a form of arthritis that affects individuals who have psoriasis (a rash that appears commonly on knees, elbows, body, and scalp and appears red and itchy with scaly patches). It is common for people to develop the rash first, followed by joint problems.

While I have an incredible amount of empathy for those who live with eczema, what I did not learn at university is that eczema and psoriasis are not even remotely the same!

There are many types of psoriasis, and an individual can have more than one type based on the symptoms. Psoriasis is also considered as an autoimmune condition where the body's immune system destroys the skin cells. The body then tries to replace this skin with new infant skin which reacts to the environment (including light, sun and air) causing intense pain. This process is constantly repeated which is why treatment is so important.

Interestingly, I continued to complain about my scalp being incredibly itchy to the point of bleeding especially at times when I was under an enormous amount of stress, particularly emotional. Having removed all gluten from my diet (even ensuring I did not get any cross contamination at all) and there were times my scalp was better managed, I still had times where the rash would erupt. This tended to lean away from the dermatitis herpetiformis being the cause. Due to this and the fact that I still continued to feel my lupus was not properly managed, I began to wonder if I had psoriatic arthritis (instead of rupus).

142

Symptoms of psoriatic arthritis, one form of psoriasis, includes swollen, painful joints that are warm to touch. Joints commonly involved include fingers, toes, hands and feet, with issues of lower back pain and foot pain. There is also a higher risk of cardiovascular health complications in those individuals with psoriatic arthritis.

On Christmas Day 2019 I woke to incredible itching on my kneecaps and outer elbow joints. So much so that I scratched them until they all bled. They were all covered in a red rash and white blisters and no number of creams or antihistamine tablets could settle the rash. I also felt totally exhausted and despite being extraordinarily busy in retail due to the time of year, this felt more to me than just end of year tiredness. Luckily, I had decided to take some time off over the holiday period because I honestly do not believe that during the following two weeks, I would have been able to work.

When I was not asleep in my bed, I was asleep on the couch or simply watching TV. That was all I could manage! While I believed that I was in a flare of my lupus, the fact that I had a rash as itchy and painful and that looked exactly what I recognised as psoriasis, I knew deep down there was more going on than I was perhaps ready to admit!

I took photos of my rash and uploaded them via email to my rheumatologist and then went and had further blood tests taken even though I knew he was on holidays. He called me immediately having seen the photos to ask how I was feeling. A quick run down and a confirmation that - you guessed it! - psoriatic arthritis was the next autoimmune condition to add to my collection! Not rheumatoid arthritis, which is more common, especially in combination with lupus. Nope, never one to be common is ME!

At least this explained why I continued to tell all my health care team I was so sore, especially (you guessed it) in my fingers, toes, feet, back, and neck. Those with psoriatic arthritis often develop pain where tendons and ligaments attach to bones. This would explain why it was always so sore to put my shoes on (especially my right foot) and why my right wrist always, always, always felt like I had broken it no matter how well I looked after it! This had been happening since 2011 and gradually getting worse! Was I happy I had another diagnosis? NO! But at least I could get treatment, now, right? Ummm maybe!

Again, despite having not been able to even really move off either the couch or my bed for almost two weeks and sleeping for almost the entire time I was on holidays, my blood results showed little out of the ordinary. So, on paper I had no inflammatory markers. Which basically meant I was unable to get the medication I needed to treat psoriatic arthritis (or lupus). Again an application was needed on compassionate grounds to the company that made one of the few medicines that could be used for both of these inflammatory conditions to see if they would give it to me free of charge (otherwise I would need to pay for it myself at about a cost of $20,000 a year because my bloods did not show I had an elevated inflammation). After nearly eight weeks' wait (which does not sound like long but is like an eternity when you are in that next level of pain constantly!) the company granted me compassionate grounds. Then after another three weeks' wait, the package arrived from the company and I was able to finally start the medicine.

The injection made me feel human again! I will always be grateful to my rheumatologist for believing in me and the symptoms I described to him. In fact, when he asked me to fill out a pain score, I had to get him to do it for me because I was unable to use a pen on the first day! Did it get my pain levels to where I expected them? NO! Was I being unrealistic in my expectations? I did not believe so! Again, pain is so very subjective that I believe it is not at all well managed at GP or specialist level! Instead of now being so fatigued that I could not work, needed to sleep all day and was unable to even perform light duties, I was now able to do basic duties but gardening, housework and a full week at work would cause such pain and fatigue that I would need two days full rest in bed. Even doubling the dose of the compassionate medicine did not seem to change my pain or fatigue score significantly!

This was despite other pain medicine that I was also taking: PEA (Palmitoylethanolamide), and CBD (cannabidiol) oil.

PEA which is produced naturally in an individual's body (and in plants and animals) is a fatty molecule that is known for its protective properties. It is known to have anti-inflammatory, anticonvulsant and pain-relieving properties and ironically is produced in lesser quantities in those who live with chronic health conditions. I do not wish to comment on PEA except to say that I found it to be effective in my own pain management.

I have written at length regarding person centred care. I find it ironic that many health care practitioners tell me they practise person centred care. The fact that health care practitioners continue to call individuals who live well with a chronic health condition a "patient" means that they really do not understand person centred care at all! To be a patient you really need to be sick, and I am NOT that! The only time this is the case is when I am admitted to hospital with something that I was unable to take care of myself! In the last twenty years I can count on one hand how many times that had happened! This did not include the times I am being proactive about my care and need to be admitted allowing for a procedure to ensure my diabetes remains well maintained with IV insulin. I was still not a patient because I was not SICK!

Person centred care also allows the person to be actively involved in the choices they make in the management of their chronic health.

This was something I found extremely difficult when I want to pursue CBD oil for my pain!

CBD is extracted from the cannabis plant (there are more than 100 compounds, collectively known as cannabinoids, derived from the plant) and has been shown to have promise in many health conditions such as chronic pain, epilepsy, cancer, multiple sclerosis and anxiety. CBD is different from THC (the compound that can make an individual high) and is thought to exert its pain-relieving effects by increasing levels of anandamide, a compound associated with regulating pain. Once again, I am not here to debate CBD. Rather I am here to comment that once I cut through layers and layers and layers and layers of red tape and was able to finally find a specialist who was comfortable to prescribe this for me, I can without a doubt say that it has helped with my pain management enormously.

So, a combination of methotrexate injection, compassionate medicine, CBD oil (at a HUGE out of pocket cost), PEA capsules and some other over the counter vitamins, was I feeling fantastic? Hardly! I feel like 100 years old most days! I am also sure there is an impact of the inflammation on my diabetes that I am aware of but could do little if anything about! I am certainly aware when I am experiencing symptoms of inflammation my glucose levels are elevated and take much longer to correct with larger doses of insulin. The resultant comment from my rheumatologist? Perhaps a pain specialist might be able to help?

I was quite at a loss to understand just how this might help given not a year or so beforehand I had already seen a pain specialist who had told me that I was "interesting but complex" and he did "not know how to help further!" When the rheumatologist made the suggestion of consulting a second pain specialist, I asked what the outcome would be, and the rheumatologist admitted he was not sure what to do next. Ahh, so finally some truth!!

As hard as this was to hear, I am ok with the truth! A second opinion in rheumatology was likely to be much more helpful at this point than one in pain management. One thing that both lupus and psoriatic arthritis have taught me over time is that I often have what I (and others) would call brain fog (it is also commonly described in studies). I have often been caught out in specialists' appointments with details, and I now carry a folder with all my details of previous results and tests. And so, armed with all my results from the last three years, this is exactly what I did! Given the recent admission that my rheumatologist was at a loss I decided it was time to drive my own health outcomes once again! While it is difficult because health literacy is not everyone's strength, it is important to ask as many questions as possible. A change in the rheumatologist also meant a change in the medicine used for the treatment of both my lupus and psoriatic arthritis (this continued on compassionate grounds because I still did not have any markers in my bloods!). The result however was an average daily pain score of 5/10; sometimes a little more, sometimes days where my pain is a little less. However, my daily fatigue is lower and my energy higher!

While I juggle a multiple of chronic health conditions every day, I am thankful for the strength it has given me. I cherish my friends and family that have always been there to support me. I am thankful for the skills I have developed as a health professional, and how I am able to negotiate the health care system for others and be able to have real conversations with people when they need it. This is what diabetes, lupus and psoriatic arthritis has taught me.

CHAPTER 20

Person (Whoops) Me Centred Care!

From the past 19 chapters, you will have seen that my road has not been straightforward. I have no doubt that you will have recognised some of the beliefs I live by. And it's those that I want to leave you with as I bring this book to a close.

The health system often talks about "patient" centred care. The very fact that the word "patient" is used in this catch phrase is ironic because it means the person using this language has simply missed the mark! If you are practising person centred care, then that person is not a patient! Unless they have been admitted to hospital and are sick!

In living with a chronic health condition, doctors and specialists interact with us approximately 1% of the time. The rest of the care and daily decision making is left to us. That is by no means a criticism, that is just reality! So really it is ME Centred Care. I am the one who makes the decisions about my health, and I should also be the one who ultimately (with guidance, support, and recommendations from my team) has the final say! Presently however this does not seem to be the way our health care system treats individuals.

To ask questions and to have an opinion, especially if that opinion differs to mainstream, an individual is most likely going to be labelled with such words as "non-compliant" or "difficult'. To do nothing about your health will certainly get you a label of "non-compliant" or now possibly the term "non adherent" or "ambivalent" because these words are deemed "softer" but mean the same thing. To "comply" with "mainstream" treatment despite obvious short falls knowing that this may cause internal conflict, has long term implications on both the mental and physical wellbeing of many individuals with chronic health issues! Sometimes you just have to keep asking questions, and not just accept a single diagnosis or what is being told to you no matter what. After all the important thing is the health and well-being of you and of your family.

In writing this book, it has not been my intention to alter the treatment of any person with a health condition because each person is totally individual in the way their body works and responds to treatments. Rather I wanted to explain how I managed the variety of responses I experienced when I used ME centred care. I improved my knowledge, my confidence and ultimately, I believe, my own health. While some health practitioners found it far too confronting, those individuals are no longer part of my team. For the members of my team that have found it refreshing and embraced it, I am eternally grateful.

For now, life has reached a good healthy equilibrium. Health and what that means is different for everyone. I will tackle whatever comes next with my team and my support as I have done in the past.

With knowledge and asking lots of questions!

www.ingramcontent.com/pod-product-compliance
Lightning Source LLC
Chambersburg PA
CBHW042247040426

42334CB00044B/3063